T0132500

Machine Learning and Deep Learning in Neuroimaging Data Analysis

Machine learning (ML) and deep learning (DL) have become essential tools in healthcare. They are capable of processing enormous amounts of data to find patterns and are also adopted into methods that manage and make sense of healthcare data, either electronic healthcare records or medical imagery. This book explores how ML/DL can assist neurologists in identifying, classifying or predicting neurological problems that require neuroimaging. With the ability to model high-dimensional datasets, supervised learning algorithms can help in relating brain images to behavioral or clinical observations and unsupervised learning can uncover hidden structures/patterns in images. Bringing together artificial intelligence (AI) experts as well as medical practitioners, these chapters cover the majority of neuro problems that use neuroimaging for diagnosis, along with case studies and directions for future research.

Anitha S. Pillai is a Professor in the School of Computing Sciences, Hindustan Institute of Technology and Science, India. She obtained a Ph.D. in the field of Natural Language Processing and has three decades of teaching/research experience. She has authored and co-authored several papers in national and international conferences/journals. She is also the Co-founder of AtINeu–Artificial Intelligence in Neurology, focusing on the applications of AI in neurological disorders.

Prof. Bindu Menon is the senior consultant neurologist, Apollo Hospitals, Nellore, Andhra Pradesh, with a teaching experience of 20 years. She has over 90 publications in various international and national journals, and has presented 100 papers and edited 2 books; she has 14 chapters to her credit. She has been conferred with a fellowship from the American Academy of Neurology, World Stroke Organization, Royal College of Physicians (Edinburg), Indian Academy of Neurology, Geriatric Society of India, Indian College of Physicians and Global Association of Physicians of Indian Origin.

She holds various positions and has several international and national awards. She is the founder of Dr. Bindu Menon Foundation and the Co-founder of AtINeu–Artificial Intelligence in Neurology.

Machine Learning and Deep Learning in Neuroimaging Data Analysis

Edited by
Anitha S. Pillai and Bindu Menon

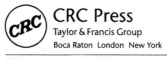

CRC Press
Taylor & Francis Group
Boca Raton London New York

CRC Press is an imprint of the
Taylor & Francis Group, an **informa** business

First edition published 2024

by CRC Press
2385 NW Executive Center Drive, Suite 320, Boca Raton FL 33431

and by CRC Press
4 Park Square, Milton Park, Abingdon, Oxon, OX14 4RN

CRC Press is an imprint of Taylor & Francis Group, LLC

Library of Congress Cataloging-in-Publication Data
Names: Pillai, Anitha S., 1967– editor. | Menon, Bindu, editor.
Title: Machine learning and deep learning in neuroimaging data analysis /
edited by Anitha S. Pillai and Bindu Menon.
Description: First edition. | Boca Raton : CRC Press, 2024. | Includes
bibliographical references. | Identifiers: LCCN 2023034284 (print) | LCCN 2023034285 (ebook) |
ISBN 9781032190686 (hbk) | ISBN 9781032207001 (pbk) | ISBN 9781003264767 (ebk)
Subjects: LCSH: Brain—Imaging—Data processing. | Artificial intelligence—Medical applications. | Neuroinformatics. |
Machine learning. | Deep learning (Machine learning)
Classification: LCC RC386.6.D52 M33 2024 (print) | LCC RC386.6.D52 (ebook) |
DDC 616.8/04754—dc23/eng/20231201
LC record available at https://lccn.loc.gov/2023034284
LC ebook record available at https://lccn.loc.gov/2023034285

ISBN: 9781032190686 (hbk)
ISBN: 9781032207001 (pbk)
ISBN: 9781003264767 (ebk)

DOI: 10.1201/9781003264767

Typeset in Minion
by codeMantra

Contents

Contributors

Ajith Abraham
Flame University, Pune, India

Dr Vikash Agarwal
SM Hospital, Assam, India

Bonny Banerjee
Institute for Intelligent Systems,
  and Department of Electrical &
  Computer Engineering, University
  of Memphis, Memphis, TN, United
  States

Lazzaro Di Biase
Fondazione Policlinico Universitario
  Campus Bio-Medico, Via Alvaro del
  Portillo, Roma, Italy

Adriano Bonura
Fondazione Policlinico Universitario
  Campus Bio-Medico, Via Alvaro del
  Portillo, Roma, Italy

Maria Letizia Caminiti
Fondazione Policlinico Universitario
  Campus Bio-Medico, Via Alvaro del
  Portillo, Roma, Italy

Subhagata Chattopadhyay
Independent Researcher, Kolkata, India

Chandra J
Christ University, Bangalore, India

Alwin Joseph
Christ University, Pune, India

Sushil S. Kokare
Garden City University, Bangalore, India

Vincenzo Di Lazzaro
Fondazione Policlinico Universitario
  Campus Bio-Medico, Via Alvaro del
  Portillo, Roma, Italy

Ms Swarna M
Clinical Research Assistant, SM Hospital,
  Assam, India

Meenakshi Malviya
Christ University, Bangalore, India

Prabha Susy Mathew
St. Francis College, Bangalore, India

Bindu Menon
Apollo Speciality Hospitals, Nellore, India

Dr. Dolly Mushahary, PhD
Clinical Research Assistant SM Hospital,
  Assam, India

Pasquale Maria Pecoraro
Fondazione Policlinico Universitario
  Campus Bio-Medico, Via Alvaro del
  Portillo, Roma, Italy

Anitha S. Pillai
Hindustan Institute of Technology and
  Science, Chennai, India

Madhavi Rangaswamy
Christ University, Bangalore, India

Jayasankara Reddy K
Christ University, Bangalore, India

Pooja V
Christ University, Bangalore, India

Revathy V. R
Garden City University, Bangalore, India

CHAPTER 1

Neuroimaging and Deep Learning in Stroke Diagnosis

A Review of a Decade of Research

Prabha Susy Mathew, Anitha S. Pillai,

Ajith Abraham, and Lazzaro Di Biase

1.1 INTRODUCTION

Globally stroke is the second leading cause of death and the third leading cause of disability. Stroke is thus a medical emergency where quick response by a medical specialist is crucial to reduce the brain damage and related complications. Early interventions can reduce brain damage and other complications. There are several risk factors that can increase the chances of one getting stroke in their lifetime. Lifestyle risk factors include being overweight or obese, physical inactivity, use of abusive substance like tobacco and alcohol. Medical risk factors include high blood pressure (BP), high cholesterol, diabetes, and family history of stroke [19]. Hypertension, also known as high blood pressure, is the most prevalent risk factor for stroke [67]. It is very important for stroke patients to understand the symptoms of stroke, as early understanding of the symptoms can lead to timely clinical interventions such as reperfusion therapy for timely care [7]. Classical symptoms include sudden weakness or numbness in the face, arm, or leg especially on one side of the body. Other symptoms include dizziness, lack of coordination, difficulty in walking or understanding speech [33]. Timely identification of the condition can prove to be very beneficial to the patient, especially in improving their clinical outcome. Early and accurate diagnosis is essential for successful treatment and enhanced outcomes in the management of stroke. The most prevalent variety of stroke is ischemic stroke (IS), which is caused by a blood clot that blocks blood flow to the brain. Early recognition and diagnosis of a stroke can limit brain damage and greatly enhance patient outcomes. In fact, early treatment of IS

DOI: 10.1201/9781003264767-1

can improve prognosis by up to 30% [36,55]. Early rehabilitation is also an essential component of stroke management, as it can enhance functional outcomes and reduce disability. Early rehabilitation, beginning within 24–48 hours of stroke onset, has been shown in clinical trials to result in improved outcomes than delayed rehabilitation. Therefore, it is essential to make an accurate and prompt diagnosis of stroke in order to initiate treatment and rehabilitation as soon as feasible.

Neuroimages such as computed tomography (CT) and magnetic resonance imaging (MRI), positron emission tomography (PET), single-photon emission tomography (SPECT), and functional MRI (fMRI), bio signals such as electrocardiogram (ECG) and Photoplethysmography (PPG) [78, 79], and electronic health records (EHR) data have been used extensively in the recent past for the disease diagnosis, prediction of clinical outcomes, and making treatment-related decisions for several disease conditions [8]. Normally, in a clinical setting, the specialist medical practitioner does the detailed interpretation of the medical images. However, interpretation of the medical images can be influenced by their level of fatigue, and the task can also get cumbersome and time-consuming. For this reason, a lot of research is being carried out to automate stroke imaging interpretations. Traditionally, machine learning (ML) algorithms were used to analyse the medical image dataset. In recent years, deep-learning (DL) algorithms have seen tremendous applications, especially in the medical image-based classification, detection, segmentation, etc., of diseases. Feature extraction, which is a very crucial part of computer vision problems, can be very efficiently carried out by DL due to its automatic feature extraction from complex image datasets [60]. Recent advances and research on ML, DL, and neuroimaging techniques have helped optimise the time-consuming tasks of detection and segmentation of the brain. It can help medical practitioners understand a patient's condition better and thereby improve their diagnosis and treatment decision-making [76].

The purpose of this review and the search strategy used to locate the research article are elaborately described in the first section. The second section discusses stroke varieties, the type of data used in stroke diagnosis, and benchmark datasets that are publicly accessible. The subsequent section focuses on the various imaging techniques used in the diagnosis of stroke. The ensuing section discusses techniques for DL. The subsequent section will emphasise clinical applications. The sixth section examines the numerous ML and DL techniques utilised for stroke diagnosis, lesion segmentation, and prognosis, among other things. Moreover, research gaps and difficulties in stroke diagnosis using DL and neuroimaging are discussed.

1.1.1 Review Objective

The following are the objectives of this review:

- To understand recent advances in DL techniques in diagnosis, prognosis, and treatment decisions for effective stroke management.

- To discuss various clinical applications of artificial intelligence (AI) techniques in stroke diagnosis and management.

- To highlight the challenges and research gaps.

1.1.2 Article Search and Selection Criteria

A comprehensive database search was conducted to identify peer-reviewed articles published between 2015 and 2022, including the following terms: 'Artificial Intelligence AND stroke', 'Ischemic Stroke', 'Acute Ischemic Stroke' (AIS), 'Hemorrhagic Stroke', 'Lesion Segmentation', 'Prognosis of Brain Strokes', 'Lesion Detection and Segmentation', and 'Neuroimaging AND Deep Learning'. Search engines used were Science Direct, Google Scholar, IEEE Xplore, Frontiers, PubMed, Springer, Wiley, and ACM.

1.2 TYPES OF STROKES

A stroke, also known as a cardiovascular accident (CVA), occurs when the blood vessel supplying oxygen and nutrients to the brain either ruptures (also known as a haemorrhagic stroke) or becomes blocked by a clot (also known as an ischemic stroke). This causes the death or damage of cerebral tissue. The *transient ischemic attack* (TIA) or *mini stroke* is a transient clot [66]. It is a temporary condition that occurs due to temporary blockage in blood flow to brain and causes no permanent brain harm. Its symptoms only last for few minutes or might continue for a couple of hours. The outcome of a stroke depends on the location of the obstruction and the extent of brain tissue injury [1]. Approximately 87% of all strokes are ischemic, while 13% are haemorrhagic. IS can be further classified as either *thrombotic stroke*, which occurs when a blood clot forms in a blood vessel within the brain, or *embolic stroke*, which occurs when a blood clot or plaque detritus from another part of the body travels to one of the brain's blood vessels. TIAs may precede the onset of a thrombotic stroke. The classification of haemorrhagic stroke [75] is as follows: High BP causes *intracerebral haemorrhage*, in which bleeding occurs unexpectedly and rapidly. It is the result of an aneurysm or an arteriovenous malformation (AVM). *Subarachnoid haemorrhage* is characterised by bleeding from the blood vessels within the brain and the membrane covering the brain in the subarachnoid space. The other categories of ICH [53] are *epidural haemorrhage* (EDH), *subdural haemorrhage* (SDH), cerebral *parenchymal haemorrhage* (CPH), and *intraventricular haemorrhage* (IVH) [65, 75] (Figure 1.1).

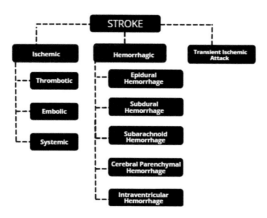

FIGURE 1.1   Stroke classification [16].

1.2.1 Data for Stroke Diagnosis

Multiple categories of data are required for the early detection of a stroke. Some important categories of data include [1].

Medical history: Information regarding a person's past medical conditions, such as a history of hypertension, diabetes, heart disease, or previous strokes, can be crucial for predicting the risk of stroke.

Lifestyle factors: Data about a person's lifestyle aspects, such as smoking, physical activity, and diet, can be crucial for predicting stroke risk. Age, gender, and ethnicity can also be significant factors in predicting the risk of stroke.

Clinical data: Data regarding BP, blood glucose levels, and cholesterol levels can reveal a lot about potential stroke risk.

Imaging studies: Imaging studies, such as MRI, CT, and ultrasound, can assist in identifying stroke risk factors, such as carotid artery disease and atrial fibrillation.

Genetic data: Genetic factors can also contribute to the risk of stroke, and genetic testing may be useful for identifying those at a higher risk.

By analysing these types of data, doctors can assess a patient's risk of suffering a stroke and devise individualised prevention strategies.

1.2.2 Some of the Publicly Available Neuroimaging Datasets

Stroke imaging is crucial in stroke management, especially when it is difficult to diagnose stroke based on clinical features. Some of the benchmark datasets that are publicly available are provided in Table 1.1.

1.3 NEUROIMAGING TECHNIQUES USED IN STROKE DIAGNOSIS

In recent years, significant research has been conducted on the role of neuroimaging in the diagnosis of stroke. Neuroimaging techniques, such as CT and MRI, are indispensable for determining the type of stroke and the extent and location of stroke-induced injury.

TABLE 1.1   Publicly available datasets for brain stroke analysis

Dataset	Number of scans	Imaging technique	References
ATLAS 2018	304	T1-weighted MR imaging	Liew et al. (2018, 2022) [39] ATLAS (nitrc.org)
ATLAS 2021	1271	T1-weighted MRIs	ATLAS (nitrc.org)
CQ500	491	CT scan	Chilamkurthy et al. [12] http://headctstudy.qure.ai/dataset
RSNA Brain Haemorrhage CT dataset	874,035	CT scan	Flanders et al. [2] https://www.rsna.org/education/ai-resources-and-training/ai-image-challenge/RSNA-Intracranial-Hemorrhage-Detection-Challenge-2019
IS lesion segmentation (ISLES) 2015–2018, 2022	150	DWI, ADC, CTP, T1-weighted MRIs	Lundervold and Lundervold (2019) [41] ISLES: Ischemic Stroke Lesion Segmentation Challenge 2015 (isles-challenge.org)

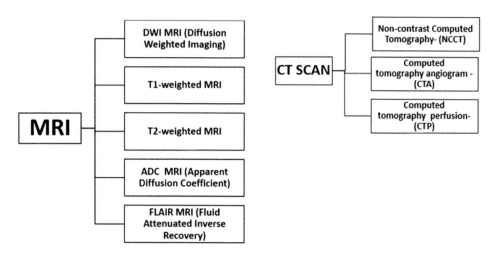

FIGURE 1.2   Types of imaging modalities in stroke diagnosis.

Understanding the pathogenesis of acute stroke and making timely and appropriate clinical decisions requires the use of modern imaging tools and techniques for the brain and its supplying blood vessels [43]. The objective of neuroimaging in the diagnosis of a stroke is to visualise the earliest phases of the development of cerebral ischemia. Diverse forms of computerised support are frequently impacted by the presence of numerous erroneous over-interpretation regions; therefore, it is of utmost importance to provide neurologically verified regions to improve the accuracy of ischemia assessment [29] (Figure 1.2).

According to recent research articles, the following neuroimaging techniques are used to diagnose stroke:

Computed tomography (CT): CT is a widely employed neuroimaging method that can promptly identify the affected vascular region of the brain in stroke patients [30]. CT can also help differentiate between stroke and its imitators, such as migraine and epilepsy [21]. Non-contrast computed tomography (NCCT) is the most commonly used first-line imaging instrument for stroke because it is simple to acquire, widely available, and effective at distinguishing between ischemia and haemorrhage. Prior to administering rtPA (recombinant tissue-type plasminogen activator) to eligible patients, it is used to rule out haemorrhage and is more accessible and less expensive than an MRI [14]. However, its ability to detect IS is inferior to that of MRI, and it exposes the patient to radiation [44].

CT angiography (CTA): CTA is an additional method for visualising blood vessels that can provide additional data on blood flow and perfusion [43].

CT perfusion: CT perfusion is a specialised neuroimaging technique that evaluates the brain's blood flow to determine if a specific brain region is receiving an adequate blood supply. CT perfusion can differentiate between ischemic and haemorrhagic strokes and determine the extent and severity of brain damage. CT perfusion is also useful for identifying common mimics of stroke, such as migraine and epilepsy perfusion imaging, using either computed tomography (CT) or MRI, and is a crucial tool in the management of stroke patients. It measures how quickly and efficiently intravenous contrast passes through specific brain regions, helping identify the ischemic core and penumbra in stroke patients. This information is vital as it can guide treatment decisions even outside the traditionally recommended treatment window.

Two key recent studies, DAWN and DEFUSE 3, used perfusion imaging to select patients for mechanical thrombectomy (MT), and reported improved patient outcomes. The primary role of this technique in AIS is to identify brain tissue that is hypoperfused (underperfused with blood) and hence at risk of infarction [51, 2]. The EXTEND (Extending the Time for Thrombolysis in Emergency Neurological Deficits) experiment has demonstrated that patients who are chosen using perfusion CT or perfusion MRI benefit from treatment with intravenous tPA up to nine hours after the start of symptoms or after a wake-up stroke [21]. This suggests that CT perfusion can be an effective strategy for extending the treatment window for patients with AIS past the usual time frame. This finding supports the use of CT perfusion in the assessment and decision-making processes for AIS patients, particularly when they present outside of the typical therapeutic time frame [56].

MRI: MRI can help identify ischemic and haemorrhagic strokes, as well as the severity of the brain injury and the vascular lesion responsible for the stroke. MRI is a technique for visualising the fundamental morphology of the brain. T1- and T2-weighted sequences detect IS more sensitively and with greater anatomical clarity than CT [59].

Diffusion-weighted imaging (DWI): DWI is used to detect small and early infarcts and to determine the suitability of endovascular therapy, but it can yield false-negative results on occasion. DW-MRI is a common stroke diagnosis technique. It can assist in distinguishing between ischemic and haemorrhagic stroke [43]. It is especially useful for the detection of acute ischemic lesions.

Perfusion-weighted imaging (PWI): PWI is used to visualise the cerebral ischemic penumbra and infarct core and to measure blood flow and functional outcome post-therapy [59].

FLAIR: FLAIR (fluid-attenuated inversion recovery) is used to detect subarachnoid haemorrhage and provides an outstanding contrast between grey and white matter lesions. Functional magnetic resonance imaging (fMRI) is used to examine the functional anatomy of the brain and assess stroke treatment and recovery.

The assessment of ischemia lesions in the brain is greatly aided by FLAIR sequences and DWI. When the moment of the stroke's onset is unknown, FLAIR sequences are particularly helpful in guiding treatment choices [6].

Magnetic resonance angiography (MRA): MRA is a non-invasive neuroimaging technique that uses MRI technology to visualise the brain's blood vessels. It is less painful, less invasive, and less expensive, and it does not expose the patient to radiation, unlike catheter angiography. MRA can identify stenosis or occlusion in the cerebral arteries and assess blood flow in the brain, thereby aiding in the diagnosis and treatment planning for stroke. The acquisition period is also longer than with CTA [30].

These methods are routinely employed in clinical practice and are essential for informing treatment decisions and enhancing patient outcomes.

In general, *multimodal neuroimaging* refers to the integration of data from various sources. It has several advantages over unimodal neuroimaging, including higher spatial and temporal resolution, the provision of more comprehensive information regarding neural processes, structures, and normalisation, and the elimination of their limitations. Thus, multimodal neuroimaging can play a significant role in disease detection, diagnosis, prognosis, and treatment [64]. PET, cerebral angiography, computed tomography angiography (CT-A), MRI, and MRA are essential imaging techniques for diagnosing intracranial haemorrhage [5]. It has been discovered that MRI DWI provides a more accurate diagnosis of AIS than a CT scan image. It is the gold standard for the detection of ISs. On the other hand, CT scan images are readily available and less expensive than MRI images [50].

1.4 DL AND ITS POTENTIAL IN STROKE DIAGNOSIS

DL is a subset of ML, which is a subset of AI. It is a technique for teaching neural networks with multiple layers to recognise and learn data patterns [13]. DL technology has demonstrated efficacy in numerous fields, including computer vision, image recognition, natural language processing, and radiology [27]. Utilising real-time biosignals and medical imaging data, DL has shown tremendous promise in stroke diagnosis for predicting and detecting stroke.

Multiple studies have documented the effective application of DL to the diagnosis of stroke. For instance, a study proposed a stroke disease prediction system utilising DL and real-time bio signals. The system was trained on a large dataset of electroencephalogram (EEG) signals and demonstrated high accuracy in stroke prediction [13]. Another study used a DL model trained on a dataset of cardiac diseases to predict stroke. The model demonstrated high sensitivity and specificity for predicting stroke, especially in patients with symptoms of atrial fibrillation [9]. DL has demonstrated tremendous promise for the diagnosis of strokes using real-time biosignals and medical imaging data. With additional research and development, DL could become a useful instrument for detecting and preventing strokes. A large number of images, such as MRI, CT, and X-ray images, are created every day. Using ML algorithms to localise such medical images is inefficient and time-consuming. Object detection using a technique based on DL can reduce the time and effort required for image inspection and evaluation. Several stroke localisation and classification methods, including R-CNN (region-based convolutional neural network), fast R-CNN (fast region-based convolutional neural network), faster R-CNN (fast region-based convolutional neural network with region proposal network), YOLO (you only look once), SSD (single-shot multibox detector), and Efficient-Det, are efficient.

1.4.1 Overview of Different DL Models Used in Stroke Diagnosis

Given the severity of the disease and the brief window of opportunity for treatment, it is crucial that a stroke be identified promptly during the initial examination. DL techniques have revolutionised the field of stroke diagnosis, leading to the development of more precise and effective diagnostic tools. These advancements have facilitated the development of new algorithms for stroke diagnosis and prognosis, thereby augmenting the clinical application of ML tools. The following are examples of common stroke diagnosis algorithms:

Convolutional neural networks (CNNs): CNNs have been shown to be effective in neuroimaging data processing, particularly in image segmentation and classification tasks. They can be used to assess characteristics such as brain structure and cortical thickness. In their work, Nugroho et al. implemented the CNN5 architectural design, which was determined to be the most effective for classifying IS, with an accuracy of 99.86%, precision of 99.862%, recall of 99.1%, and F1 score of 99.86% [52].

Recurrent neural networks (RNNs): RNNs have demonstrated promise in the processing of time-series data, including EEG and fMRI signals. They can be utilised to examine features such as brain connectivity and functional networks. A three-dimensional joint CNN-RNN DL framework was developed to accurately detect ICH and its subtypes, with the potential to reduce misinterpretations [75].

Support vector machines (SVMs): SVMs are a ML algorithm that has been applied to neuroimaging data in several investigations. They can be utilised to analyse characteristics such as regional brain volumes and patterns of brain activation. In their study, Al-Mekhlafi et al. compared the efficacy of the AlexNet model and the AlexNet + SVM hybrid technique for early detection of stroke and haemorrhage using an MRI dataset. AlexNet + SVM outperformed AlexNet; it obtained 99.9% accuracy, 100% sensitivity, 99.80% specificity, and 99.86% area under the curve (AUC) [3].

Long short-term memory (LSTM): The LSTM RNN is intended for the management of long-term dependencies. EEG signals can be modelled using them. Yu et al. designed and implemented a stroke disease prediction system that integrates CNN and LSTM into an ensemble structure to predict stroke disease in real-time while strolling. Their model employed ECG and PPG biosignals sampled at 1,000 Hz from the three ECG electrodes and the index finger for PPG. Their CNN-LSTM model's prediction accuracy of 99.15% was commendable [78]. Another study utilising EEG sensor data compared various DL models (LSTM, bidirectional LSTM (B-LSTM), CNN-LSTM, and CNN-bidirectional LSTM), and their findings confirmed that the CNN-bidirectional LSTM model, when applied to unprocessed EEG data, could accurately predict stroke with a 94.0% accuracy rate [13].

Autoencoders are a type of neural network that can be used for unsupervised feature learning. One study used an autoencoder to detect anomalies in brain connection data, which may be useful for early stroke detection [58]. Using multimodal MRI data, another study proposed a novel autoencoder-LSTM model for predicting the prognosis of a stroke, which can be beneficial for stroke management [57]. In another study, the authors proposed a prediction model for IS based on ECG signals and B-LSTM. The model aims to improve the early detection and diagnosis of IS, which can facilitate the prompt implementation of treatment. The study demonstrates that the proposed B-LSTM model is 92% accurate at predicting IS [35].

1.4.2 Performance Analysis of DL Models on Benchmark Datasets

Several publicly available benchmark datasets have been used by researchers for diagnosis of stroke. Some of the most recent work using DL approaches with a range of performance metrics, such as accuracy, Dice coefficient, and F1 score, have been shown in the Table 1.2.

Notably, a hybrid AlexNet and SVM model achieved an average accuracy of 99.86% on a Kaggle dataset, while other models like U-Net-based CNN and VGG16-SegNet demonstrated promising results on the ISLES 2015 MRI imaging data and ATLAS (Anatomical Tracings of Lesions After Stroke) dataset (Figure 1.3).

TABLE 1.2   Performance analysis of DL models on publicly available benchmark datasets

S.No	Studies	Method	Outcome	Benchmark MRI dataset
1	Xue et al. (2019)	3D asymmetrical encoder-decoder network based on the U-Net	Dice coefficient –0.62	Medical College of Wisconsin (MCW), Kessler Foundation (KF), and the publicly available ATLAS dataset
2	Lui et al. (2019)	Multi-kernel DCNN	Dice coefficient of 0.57	ISLES 2015
3	Gaidhani (2019)	LeNet for classification and auto encoder-decoder for segmentation	Classification accuracy:0.98Precsion:0.97Recall-0.97 F1 score 0.97 Segmentation accuracy: 0.85	ATLAS
4	Karthick et al. (2020)	Multi-level Return on Investment-aligned deconvolutional ensemble	Dice coefficient of 0.775	ISLES 2015
5	Rajinikanth et al. (2021)	VGG16-SegNet	Accuracy: 97	ISLES 2015
6	Al-Mekhlafi et al. (2021)	AlexNet	Accuracy: 96.8 Precision: 97 Sensitivity: 96.7 Specificity: 96.9 AUC: 96.8	https://www.kaggle.com/abdulkader90/brain-ct-hemorrhage-dataset
7	Al-Mekhlafi et al. (2021)	Hybrid AlexNet + SVM	Accuracy: 99.9, Precision: 100, Sensitivity: 100 Specificity: 99.8 AUC: 99.86	https://www.kaggle.com/abdulkader90/brain-ct-hemorrhage-dataset
8	Barin et al. (2021)	Hybrid EfficientNet-B3 and ResNet-Inception-V2	Accuracy: 98.6 Precision: 91.2 Sensitivity: 83.1 Specificity: 99.5 AUC: 1	RSNA Intracranial Hemorrhage Detection	Kaggle
9	Clérigues et al. (2021)	U-Net based CNN	SISS (DSC=0.59 ± 0.31) SPES sub-tasks (DSC=0.84 ± 0.10)	ISLES 2015

1.5 APPLICATIONS OF NEUROIMAGING AND DL IN STROKE DIAGNOSIS

Some of the clinical applications of AI for stroke diagnosis are given below.

1.5.1 Classification of Stroke

Numerous studies have investigated the use of DL algorithms for stroke classification in recent years. Utilising transfer learning and hyperparameter optimisation, Chen et al. created a DL-based method for classifying cerebral CT images of stroke patients. CNN-based DL models were implemented for efficient classification of strokes based on unenhanced brain CT images into normal, haemorrhage, and other categories. With an accuracy of 0.9872, the CNN-2 and ResNet-50 outperformed the VGG-16, according to the results [11]. Nugroho et al. classified IS using a CNN approach on b-1000 diffusion-weighted magnetic resonance imaging (DW-MRI) and achieved a 99.86% classification accuracy [52]. In neuroradiology, Dawud et al. classified cerebral haemorrhages using transfer learning and DL [15]. Zhu and coworkers presented a dataset for stroke classification in electromagnetic imaging utilising novel graph-degree mutual information (GDMI) approaches to distinguish intracranial haemorrhage (ICH) from IS with 88% accuracy (Zhu et al., 2021). Marbun et al. used CNN to classify stroke diseases [42]. Gautam and Raman used CNN on CT scan images to devise an effective classification method for haemorrhagic and ischemic brain injuries. The robustness of the method was determined by undertaking two experiments on two distinct datasets. Comparing the outcomes of the proposed method to those of AlexNet and ResNet50 revealed that the proposed model produced superior results [22]. The study by Yalcn and Vural, titled "Brain stroke classification and segmentation using U-Net, encoder-decoder-based deep convolutional neural networks", focuses on

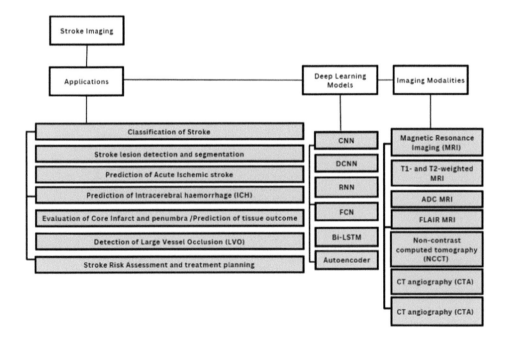

FIGURE 1.3   DL learning on stroke imaging.

the application of deep CNNs for the classification and segmentation of brain stroke using CT scan images. The study proposes an encoder-decoder CNN architecture that extracts features from input images using an encoder network and reconstructs the output image using a decoder network. The model achieved a 98.9% accuracy for stroke classification and a 95.5% intersection over union (IoU) rate for segmentation [73]. In another study, authors assessed the efficacy of a novel three-dimensional joint convolutional and recurrent neural network (CNN-RNN) for the detection of intracranial haemorrhage (ICH) and its five sub-types (cerebral parenchymal, intraventricular, subdural, epidural, and subarachnoid) in non-contrast head CT. The researchers trained and evaluated their model using a dataset containing 4,396 ICH patients and 4,949 healthy controls. The efficacy of the model was evaluated by comparing it to the standard two-dimensional CNN model and the radiologists' diagnoses. The outcomes demonstrated that the three-dimensional joint CNN-RNN model outperformed the conventional two-dimensional CNN model and obtained a high level of precision in detecting ICH and its subtypes. The model exhibited an area under the curve (AUC) of 0.987 for the detection of ICH and AUCs of 0.972 for other analytes [75].

1.5.2 Stroke Detection and Segmentation

In recent years, neuroimaging and DL techniques have made substantial advancements in the detection and segmentation of stroke lesions. These techniques have been applied to the development of more precise, efficient, and automated systems for the analysis of medical images associated with strokes, thereby facilitating diagnosis and prognosis.

Medical imaging, stroke diagnosis, and treatment all depend on the segmentation of ischemic or haemorrhagic lesions. It provides for precise localisation and measurement of the size of the lesion, as well as longitudinal study, increased reproducibility, and research support. CNNs and other automated techniques for segmenting ischemic or haemorrhagic lesions have been developed as a result of recent developments in DL and AI. The effectiveness and speed of stroke diagnosis can be increased considerably by using these techniques [63]. Karthik et al. provide a comprehensive overview of recent advancements and future prospects in neuroimaging and DL for detecting cerebral strokes in their study. This study investigates the impact of DL models on cerebral stroke detection and lesion segmentation, with a focus on the most recent approaches proposed in the field [33].

Han et al. proposed an Internet of Medical Things (IoMT)-based method for segmentation of lung and stroke regions in CT scans using DL. This article discusses the application of DL techniques to segment lung and stroke regions in CT images. The paper emphasises the significance of classification and segmentation of pathologies using intelligent systems for medical image analysis and computer vision systems [24]. Hu et al. presented BrainSegNet, a residual three-dimensional framework for the automatic segmentation of lesions from perfusion MR images obtained from the Ischemic Stroke Lesion Segmentation (ISLES) 2017 database [26]. Another study proposed a multi-path, 2.5-dimensional CNN system for segmenting stroke lesions in MRI images of the brain [72]. Karthik et al. (2021) proposed an ensemble of multi-scale, region-aligned deep architectures based on fully convolutional networks (FCNs) and cascaded CNNs for the segmentation of ischemic lesions. On the ISLES 2015 dataset, the model was evaluated, and a mean dice coefficient of 0.77

was attained [32]. Wu et al. proposed a novel data augmentation strategy for a DL-based neuroimaging segmentation method. The conditional generative adversarial network (cGAN) and supervised CNN segmentation were used to generate additional MRI images from specially modified masks, and the method was evaluated using the ATLAS dataset [71]. Using CNNs, Woo et al. proposed a completely automatic method for segmenting acute ischemic lesions on DWI with Dice indices greater than or equal to 0.85 and found the approach to be superior to traditional algorithms [70].

DL models, in particular CNNs, have been applied to various aspects of stroke detection and segmentation, such as the classification of distinct categories of strokes and the identification of the location and extent of brain lesions. These models can autonomously extract abstract features for classification, detection, and segmentation from a large number of samples, thereby facilitating the intelligent interpretation of MRI scans. In their investigation, three types of DL object detection networks, namely, faster R-CNN, YOLOV3, and SSD, were employed to implement automatic lesion detection with 89.77% accuracy [82]. For detecting and segmenting haemorrhagic strokes in CT brain images, a U-net-based method is an example of a DL framework [37]. This method addresses the issue of high variability in stroke location, contrast, and morphology, which can be challenging for experienced radiologists to identify. In their paper, Zhang Y et al. examined various DL algorithms applied to publicly accessible datasets, including ISLES 2015, 2017, and 2018, and the ATLAS dataset. Although DL techniques have been widely used in medical image lesion segmentation, it remains challenging to apply these techniques to segment IS lesions due to differences in lesion characteristics, segmentation difficulty, algorithm maturity, and segmentation accuracy compared to brain tumours [83].

Hssayeni et al. proposed a deep convolutional model for intracranial haemorrhage (ICH) segmentation in CT images. The objective of the study was to develop a precise and effective DL model to assist clinicians in diagnosing ICH and determining the extent of the haemorrhage. The authors developed their model using a modified U-Net architecture, a prominent DL model for image segmentation tasks. They trained and validated the model using 197 CT scans with ICH and more than 9,000 axial slices from a dataset containing over 9,000 slices. The efficacy of the model was measured using sensitivity, specificity, and the Dice similarity coefficient (DSC). The outcomes demonstrated that the proposed deep convolutional model achieved promising segmentation results. The model attained 77.1% sensitivity, 99.5% specificity, and a DSC of 0.74. These results suggest that the proposed model has the potential to serve as an effective instrument for segmenting ICH in CT images, thereby enhancing the diagnosis and treatment planning for patients with ICH [25].

For detecting and segmenting IS lesions using DL networks, the authors developed a tool. The tool was trained and evaluated on a dataset of 2,348 clinical diffusion-weighted MRIs of patients with acute and sub-AIS, and its generalisation was evaluated on an external dataset of 280 MRIs. The proposed model three-dimensional network, called DAGMNet, outperforms generic networks such as U-Net, FCN, and DeepMedic. The tool is quick, open-source, accessible to non-experts, requires minimal computation, and can detect and segment lesions with a single command line [40]. Large vessel occlusion (LVO) refers to the obstruction of large, proximal cerebral arteries in the brain, which may account for up to 46% of AIS. LVO detection is crucial for timely treatment and enhanced outcomes in patients with AIS. Here are some recent studies concerning the detection of LVO [82]. Kamnitsas et al. demonstrated the capability of a three-dimensional CNN for the automated detection of AIS on multimodal MRI scans. The authors utilised a CNN architecture with multiple scales and trained it on two large publicly available benchmark datasets, BRATS 2015 and ISLES 2015 of MRI scans. The model outperformed conventional ML methods in detecting AIS lesions, yielding optimistic results [31].

You J et al. proposed three hierarchical models to increase the accuracy and efficiency of identifying LVO in patients with AIS by combining demographic, clinical, and CT scan features. Their third model extracted features from CT scan images using DL. Multiple ML techniques, including logistic regression, random forest, SVM, and eXtreme Gradient Boosting (XGboost), were utilised in the modelling of all three levels [81, 82]. Nishi et al. designed a multioutput CNN model for segmentation of the ischemic core lesion for the extraction of high-level imaging features and prediction of the long-term clinical outcome. The architecture for segmentation was based on U-Net. The authors used DL to derive imaging features from pre-treatment DWI data and evaluated these features' ability to predict clinical outcomes for patients with LVO. Models' performances were internally validated with five-fold cross-validation using the standard neuroimaging biomarkers Alberta Stroke Programme Early CT (ASPECT) score and volume of ischemic core. The AUC was found to be substantially superior during external validation of the CNN model [49]. ICH is a condition associated with a high incidence of morbidity and mortality and is life-threatening. It is a potentially fatal condition characterised by bleeding within the brain tissue. Recent research has focused on the development of predictive models to identify patients at high risk of ICH, enabling earlier intervention and improving outcomes.

In research conducted by Chilamkurthy et al., they demonstrated that a CNN can effectively detect ICH on head CT scans. The authors trained their CNN on a large dataset of anonymised head CT scans and obtained an AUC of 0.91, indicating high diagnostic accuracy [12]. Grewal et al. proposed a 40-layer CNN with a B-LSTM layer for ICH detection, with 81% accuracy, 88% recall, 81% precision, and an 84% F1 score [23].

Software solutions are available to aid in the detection and measurement of the ischemic core and penumbra in patients who have experienced a stroke. Examples include RAPID (iSchemaView), Aidoc, Avicenna.AI, Viz CTP (Viz.ai), and e-CTP (Brainomix) [61].

RAPID (iSchemaView) is a cutting-edge neuroimaging technology that helps with real-time processing of brain images for evaluation of stroke.

Aidoc provides a sophisticated AI platform utilised in the general identification and evaluation of stroke.

Avicenna.AI provides solutions for the diagnosis and treatment of strokes.

Viz.ai is a solution that analyses brain scans and looks for strokes that may have been caused by suspected major vessel occlusions.

e-CTP (Brainomix) is a tool employed in the evaluation of CT perfusion imagery. It helps doctors make decisions about acute stroke therapy by providing precise maps and measurements of the ischemic core and penumbra.

1.5.3 Prediction of Stroke

Arterial ischemic stroke occurs when an obstructed artery prevents blood from reaching a portion of the brain, resulting in cell death and brain tissue loss. Detection and intervention at an early stage are essential for reducing the risk of disability or mortality. Recent advances in DL algorithms and neuroimaging techniques have demonstrated promise for the early detection and forecasting of AIS. The authors in their study constructed and validated DL models based on multiparametric MRI to automatically predict haemorrhagic transformation (HT) in patients with AIS. The models incorporated multiparametric MRI and clinical data of AIS patients with endovascular thrombectomy (EVT) from two centres. The DWI, MTT, TTP, and clinical (DMTC) model performed the best at predicting HT, with an accuracy of 94%. The proposed clinical, DWI, and PWI multiparameter DL model has the potential to aid in the periprocedural management of AIS [28]. Another study examines the application of DL to predict the underlying mechanisms of AIS using MRI data from the brain. The authors use a CNN model to identify the mechanism of a stroke from MRI images, which can aid in providing personalised treatment and improving patient outcomes. The study demonstrates the potential for DL techniques to improve stroke diagnosis and treatment [54]. In another study, the authors developed a deep neural network (DNN) model to predict final IS lesions from initial DWI. The objective of their study was to enhance the prognosis and treatment planning for stroke patients by accurately estimating the infarct's final volume and location. To predict ultimate infarct volume and location in acute stroke patients, the authors employed an attention-gated (AG) DCNN model trained with DWI obtained at admission. This approach has the potential to enhance patient outcomes and facilitate clinical decision-making. Their model obtained an AUC of 0.91 [45].

The mortality rate associated with hemotome expansion in spontaneous ICH is among the highest in neurosurgery. Tang et al. propose a method for predicting hematoma expansion (HE) in spontaneous ICH from brain CT imaging. It uses K-nearest neighbours matting to remove the outer portion of the cranium and preserve brain tissue features and a deep residual network to learn from hematoma and other brain tissue characteristics. The proposed framework can achieve superior prediction performance using only brain CT scans [62].

In another similar study, the authors implemented a DL approach that replicates the interpretation process of radiologists by combining a two-dimensional CNN model with two sequence models to detect and classify ICH subtypes accurately. The extensive 2019-RSNA Brain CT Haemorrhage Challenge dataset, containing over 25,000 CT scans, was utilised to develop the DL algorithm. With AUCs of 0.988 (ICH), 0.984 (EDH), 0.992 (IPH), 0.996 (IVH), 0.985 (SAH), and 0.983 (SDH), the algorithm accurately classified acute ICH and its five subtypes, reaching expert radiologist accuracy. The authors' method won first place in the RSNA (Radiological Society of North America) challenge among 1345 teams from 75 countries. The algorithm was further evaluated on two independent external validation datasets containing 75 and 491 CT scans, maintaining high AUCs for acute ICH detection of 0.964% and 0.949%, respectively [68]. Pérez del Barrio et al. developed a DL model to predict prognosis following intracranial haemorrhage (ICH). The objective was to create an accurate and efficient method for determining the clinical outcomes of patients with ICH, which could facilitate personalised treatment planning and improve patient care. Their model obtained an AUC-ROC of 0.91, 85.4% accuracy, 88.1% sensitivity, and intracranial haemorrhage (ICH). The objective was to create an accurate and efficient method for determining the clinical outcomes of patients with ICH, which could facilitate personalised treatment planning and improve patient care. Their model obtained an AUC-ROC of 0.91, 85.4% accuracy, 88.1% sensitivity, and 82.3% specificity, respectively.

1.5.4 Evaluation of Core Infarct and Penumbra/Prediction of Tissue Outcome

During an AIS, the core infarct refers to the region of the brain that has endured infarction or is destined to infarct irreversibly regardless of reperfusion. The ischemic penumbra, on the other hand, is the component of an AIS that is susceptible to infarction but still salvageable if reperfused [33]. The penumbra is typically located around the infarct's nucleus and represents blood-depleted tissue. The primary objective of acute stroke intervention is to restore blood flow and reperfuse the affected region in order to halt the progression of the penumbra to irreversible infarction. Existing studies on MRI and CT perfusion imaging are able to precisely quantify the infarct core and penumbra, thereby guiding treatment decisions and predicting patient outcomes.

Winder et al. proposed a modular UNet-based deep convolutional network (DCN) for predicting follow-up lesions in AIS patients using baseline CT perfusion (CTP) datasets. Temporal feature extraction is separated from tissue outcome prediction in the model, enabling model validation using perfusion parameter maps and end-to-end learning from spatiotemporal CTP data. This strategy has the potential to enhance clinical decision-making by providing more precise predictions of tissue outcomes in patients with AIS [69]. Using acute MRI, Yu et al. developed and trained a deep convolutional neural network (CNNdeep) to predict the ultimate imaging outcome in AIS patients. The study comprises 222 patients, 187 of whom were treated with rtPA. Using features extracted from MRI data, the efficacy of the CNNdeep model is compared to that of a shallow CNN. Such approaches could enhance patient management and treatment planning [80]. The study, "Prediction of Tissue Outcome and Assessment of Treatment Effect in Acute Ischemic Stroke Using Deep Learning", investigates the potential of DL techniques to predict tissue outcomes and assess treatment effects in patients with AIS. The authors used deep CNN to analyse MRI data from patients with AIS. Its performance was compared to shallow CNN performance using PWI. Deep CNN significantly outperformed shallow CNN in predicting the final outcome [48].

1.5.5 Stroke Risk Assessment and Treatment Planning

The application of AI technology, including DL techniques, in the assessment of stroke risk has yielded positive results [18]. DL can solve exceedingly difficult problems such as image classification, natural language processing, and drug discovery by training neural networks. These capabilities can be utilised to predict stroke risk and outcomes, providing clinicians and patients with valuable information. A study used DL algorithms, including Yolo V3, R-CNN, and MobileNet, to identify carotid plaque from MRI scans in order

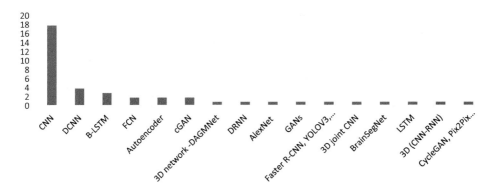

FIGURE 1.4 Different DL models used in stroke analysis discussed in this review.

to assess the risk of stroke [10]. The trained YOLO V3 model achieved an accuracy of 94.81%, the R-CNN achieved an accuracy of 92.53%, and MobileNet achieved an accuracy of 90.20%. By employing these algorithms, the study intended to prevent erroneous diagnoses resulting from poor image quality and subjective judgement. Liu et al. developed a tool based on DL that was evaluated in two clinical contexts, demonstrating its potential to improve stroke diagnosis and treatment planning. Dev et al. [17] used features of patients in EHR to make stroke predictions. They found that just four features A, HD, HT, and AG, namely (age, heart disease, hypertension, and average glucose levels) made a significant impact on stroke prediction. The neural network performed best when A, HD, HT, and AG were combined, and obtained the accuracy and miss rate of 78% and 19%, respectively (Figure 1.4).

1.6 TECHNICAL AND NON-TECHNICAL CHALLENGES IN UTILISING NEUROIMAGING AND DL FOR STROKE DIAGNOSIS AND MONITORING

Utilising neuroimaging and DL can aid in the accurate diagnosis and monitoring of a stroke, leading to improved patient outcomes. However, there are also technical and non-technical obstacles that researchers in this field must overcome.

1.6.1 Need for Large, Quality, and Varied Datasets

The need for extensive and diverse datasets is one of the technical challenges [33]. Effective training of DL models requires vast quantities of data, and stroke datasets can be limited in scale and scope. Moreover, different types of strokes (such as ischemic and haemorrhagic) can present differently on imaging; thus, it is essential to train on a diversity of cases [34]. Wu et al. in their study proposed a method of superimposition of lesion masks to increase the size of the dataset and to introduce data diversity effectively [71]. Nie et al., in their work published in 2016, used three-dimensional FCNs to generate CT brain images from MRI brain images. Reducing cost and enhancing patient safety by eliminating the need for a CT scan and the ionising radiation emitted by CT scanners. Nie et al., in 2017, utilised the capacity of generative adversarial network (GANs) to generate enhanced, higher-resolution images from native CT images. These algorithmically generated, high-quality MRI images on a lower-field-strength scanner would reduce healthcare costs [46, 47]. In a similar study, authors used DL techniques to develop a method for synthesising MRI images from brain CT images to assist in MR-guided radiotherapy. Several DL network models, including CycleGAN, the Pix2Pix model, and U-Net, were utilised to implement this brain MRI synthesis. The quantitative comparisons indicated that the performance of U-Net, a supervised DL method, was superior to that of CycleGAN, a typical unsupervised method [38].

Due to the imbalanced nature of healthcare data, its analysis can result in skewed predictions and the misclassification of severe medical conditions. Dev et al. implemented an innovative DNN technique coupled with an artificial bee colony feature selection method to improve prediction performance and ensure accurate stroke case identification. Both a ten-fold cross-validation method and a 50–50 training-testing method are used to evaluate the results, and it was discovered that the ten-fold cross-validation method yields superior results. The model achieved an accuracy rate of 87.09%, outperforming existing methods and demonstrating its applicability in the real world [16].

To address the issues of data paucity W. Wu et al. proposed a data augmentation framework using a cGAN followed by supervised segmentation with a CNN to address this problem. The cGAN generates meaningful brain images from specially modified lesion masks as a form of data augmentation to supplement the training dataset, whereas the CNN incorporates depth-wise convolution-based X-blocks and the feature similarity module (FSM) to facilitate and aid the training process, resulting in improved lesion segmentation. On the ATLAS dataset, the proposed DL strategy is evaluated and shown to outperform the current state-of-the-art algorithms for stroke lesion segmentation [2, 71]. Various strategies, such as data augmentation, transfer learning [77], GANs, and multimodal fusion frameworks, can be used to address this issue.

1.6.2 Integration of Multimodal Data

The combination of multiple imaging data types, such as MRI and CT, can provide a more complete picture of a patient's condition. However, integrating these diverse modalities can be technically challenging and necessitates specialised knowledge and methods. In multimodal neuroimaging fusion frameworks, DL models are utilised to learn feature representations of each modality and then combine them for subsequent tasks. Popular techniques include multimodal reconstruction, deep canonical correlation analysis (DCCA), and knowledge-transfer-based fusion [74].

1.6.3 Robust and Interpretable Models

Another technical challenge is the development of robust and interpretable models. DL models can be complex and difficult to interpret, making it important to develop models that can be understood by clinicians and integrated into clinical practice. Additionally, these models must be able to generalise to new cases and imaging modalities. Another related issue in neuroimaging is that the datasets can differ in terms of imaging protocols. Such variability can impact the performance of DL models, making it crucial to standardise imaging protocols and develop models that can accommodate image quality variations.

1.6.4 Lack of Sufficient Labelled Data

High mortality rates are associated with, for which the paper proposes an integrated method to enhance medical image analysis. Currently, the majority of medical image analysis for critical stroke conditions such as cerebral ischemia and intracranial haemorrhagic conditions is performed manually, which is time-consuming and labour-intensive. Lack of sufficient labelled data is one of the primary challenges in the field, which has slowed the development of DL methods.

1.6.5 Overfitting

Data augmentation and transfer learning are the two most commonly used methods for combating the overfitting problem in stroke analysis using DL and neuroimaging. Data augmentation expands neuroimaging datasets, whereas transfer learning involves pre-training a model on a large-scale dataset and refining it on a smaller, domain-specific dataset. Multi-task learning enables a model to simultaneously solve multiple related tasks, resulting in improved generalisation and less overfitting. Combining modalities, ensemble learning, regularisation and early halting, domain adaptation, and unsupervised domain adaptation are all techniques used to enhance the performance of DL models for stroke lesions [4, 33, 77].

1.6.6 Computational Resources

DL models can be computationally intensive, demanding substantial hardware and software resources. This can be a barrier to adoption, especially in settings with limited resources.

Non-technical issues include the need for specialised knowledge and methods to integrate diverse modalities and make the models accessible to clinicians. The integration of neuroimaging and DL has the potential to revolutionise the field and improve patient outcomes despite these challenges.

1.7 CONCLUSION

Neuroimaging and DL can play a crucial role in the treatment of cerebral lesions. Stroke is the leading cause of mortality and disability on a global scale, and early diagnosis and treatment are crucial for improving patient outcomes. Neuroimaging techniques, such as CT and MRI, are used to diagnose stroke and assess the severity of brain damage.

Learning algorithms can assist with the analysis of neuroimaging data and the early detection of stroke. For instance, CNNs can be used to analyse CT or MRI images of the brain in order to automatically detect stroke indicators such as ischemic lesions and haemorrhages. These algorithms can facilitate a faster and more accurate diagnosis and help physicians make informed treatment decisions.

DL can also be used to predict the outcomes of stroke patients. For instance, recurrent neural networks (RNNs) can be used to analyse longitudinal imaging data and clinical variables in order to predict outcomes such as mortality, functional disability, and cognitive impairment. Such predictions can aid in the planning and allocation of resources and treatments.

Overall, DL and neuroimaging have immense potential for improving stroke management, from early detection and diagnosis to treatment guidance and patient outcome prediction. Additional research can aid in the creation of more precise and individualised stroke management strategies.

REFERENCES

1. About Stroke | American Stroke Association. (n.d.). American Stroke Association. Retrieved October 7, 2022, from https://www.stroke.org/en/about-stroke
2. Albers, G. W., Marks, M. P., Kemp, S., et al. (2018). Thrombectomy for Stroke at 6 to 16 Hours with Selection by Perfusion Imaging. *The New England Journal of Medicine*, 378(8), 708–718.
3. Al-Mekhlafi, Z. G., Senan, E. M., Rassem, T. H., Mohammed, B. A., Makbol, N. M., Alanazi, A. A., Almurayziq, T. S., & Ghaleb, F. A. (2022). Deep Learning and Machine Learning for Early Detection of Stroke and Haemorrhage. *Computers, Materials and Continua*, 72(1), 775–796. https://doi.org/10.32604/cmc.2022.024492
4. Avberšek, L. K., & Repovš, G. (2022). Deep Learning in Neuroimaging Data Analysis: Applications, Challenges, and Solutions.
5. Barin, S., Saribaş, M., Çiltaş, B. G., Güraksin, G. E., & Köse, U. (2021). Hybrid Convolutional Neural Network-Based Diagnosis System for Intracranial Hemorrhage. BRAIN. *Broad Research in Artificial Intelligence and Neuroscience*, 12(4), 01–27. https://doi.org/10.18662/brain/12.4/236
6. Benzakoun, J., Deslys, M. A., Legrand, L., Hmeydia, G., Turc, G., Hassen, W. B., Charron, S., Debacker, C., Naggara, O., Baron, J. C., Thirion, B., Oppenheim, C. (2022 April) Synthetic FLAIR as a Substitute for FLAIR Sequence in Acute Ischemic Stroke. *Radiology*, 303(1):153–159. https://doi.org/10.1148/radiol.211394. Epub 2022 Jan 11. PMID: 35014901.
7. Bull Iversen, A., Blauenfeldt, R. A., Johnsen, S. P., Sandal, B. F., Christensen, B., Andersen, G., & Christensen, M. B. (2022). Understanding the Seriousness of a Stroke Is Essential for Appropriate Help-Seeking and Early Arrival at a Stroke Centre: A Cross-sectional Study of Stroke Patients and Their Bystanders. *European Stroke Journal 2020*, 5(4), 351–361. Sage Publication. https://doi.org/10.1177/2396987320945834
8. Castillo, D., Lakshminarayanan, V., & Rodríguez-Álvarez, M. J. (2021). Mr Images, Brain Lesions, and Deep Learning. *Applied Sciences (Switzerland)*, 11(4), 1–41. https://doi.org/10.3390/app11041675
9. Chantamit-O-Pas, P., & Goyal, M. (2017). Prediction of Stroke Using Deep Learning Model. Lecture Notes in Computer Science (Including Subseries Lecture Notes in Artificial Intelligence and Lecture Notes in Bioinformatics), 10638 LNCS, 774–781. https://doi.org/10.1007/978-3-319-70139-4_78
10. Chen, Y. F., Chen, Z. J., Lin, Y. Y., Lin, Z. Q., Chen, C. N., Yang, M. L., Zhang, J. Y., Li, Y. Z., Wang, Y., & Huang, Y. H. (2023). Stroke Risk Study Based on Deep Learning-Based Magnetic Resonance Imaging Carotid Plaque Automatic Segmentation Algorithm. Frontiers in Cardiovascular Medicine, 10. https://doi.org/10.3389/fcvm.2023.1101765
11. Chen, Y. T., Chen, Y. L., Chen, Y. Y., Huang, Y. T., Wong, H. F., Yan, J. L., & Wang, J. J. (2022). Deep Learning-Based Brain Computed Tomography Image Classification with Hyperparameter Optimization through Transfer Learning for Stroke. *Diagnostics*, 12(4).
12. Chilamkurthy, S., Ghosh, R., Tanamala, S., Biviji, M., Campeau, N. G., Venugopal, V. K., Mahajan, V., Rao, P., & Warier, P. (2018). Deep Learning Algorithms for Detection of Critical Findings in Head CT Scans: A Retrospective Study. *The Lancet*, 392(10162), 2388–2396. https://doi.org/10.1016/S0140-6736(18)31645-3
13. Choi, Y. A., Park, S. J., Jun, J. A., Pyo, C. S., Cho, K. H., Lee, H. S., & Yu, J. H. (2021). Deep Learning-Based Stroke Disease Prediction System Using Real-Time Bio Signals. *Sensors*, 21(13). https://doi.org/10.3390/s21134269

14. Czap, A. L., & Sheth, S. A. (2021). Overview of Imaging Modalities in Stroke. *Neurology*, 97(20 Supplement 2), S42–S51. https://doi.org/10.1212/WNL.0000000000012794

15. Dawud, A. M., Yurtkan, K., & Oztoprak, H. (2019). Application of Deep Learning in Neuroradiology: Brain Haemorrhage Classification Using Transfer Learning. *Computational Intelligence and Neuroscience*, 2019. https://doi.org/10.1155/2019/4629859

16. Dev, A., & Malik, S. K. (2021). Artificial Bee Colony Optimized Deep Neural Network Model for Handling Imbalanced Stroke Data: ABC-DNN for Prediction of Stroke. *International Journal of E-Health and Medical Communications*, 12(5), 67–83. https://doi.org/10.4018/IJEHMC.20210901.oa5

17. Dev, S., Wang, H., Nwosu, C. S., Jain, N., Veeravalli, B., & John, D. (2022, November). A Predictive Analytics Approach for Stroke Prediction Using Machine Learning and Neural Networks. *Healthcare Analytics*, 2, 100032. https://doi.org/10.1016/j.health.2022.100032

18. Ding, L., Liu, C., Li, Z., & Wang, Y. (2020). Incorporating Artificial Intelligence into Stroke Care and Research. *Stroke*, 51(12), E351–E354. https://doi.org/10.1161/STROKEAHA.120.031295

19. Dr Poonam Khetrapal Singh. (2021). World Stroke Day. https://www.who.int/southeastasia/news/detail/28-10-2021-world-stroke-day

20. El-Wahsh, S., Dunkerton, S., Ang, T., Winters, H. S., & Delcourt, C. (2021). Current Perspectives on Neuroimaging Techniques Used to Identify Stroke Mimics in Clinical Practice. In *Expert Review of Neurotherapeutics* (Vol. 21, Issue 5, pp. 517–531). Taylor and Francis Ltd. https://doi.org/10.1080/14737175.2021.1911650

21. Flanders, A. E. Prevedello, L. M., Shih, G. et al. (2020). Construction of a Machine Learning Dataset through Collaboration: The RSNA 2019 Brain CT Hemorrhage Challenge. *Radiology: Artificial Intelligence*, 2, 3.

22. Gautam, A., & Raman, B. (2021). Towards Effective Classification of Brain Hemorrhagic and Ischemic Stroke Using CNN. *Biomedical Signal Processing and Control*, 63. https://doi.org/10.1016/j.bspc.2020.102178

23. Grewal, M., Srivastava, M. M., Kumar, P., & Varadarajan, S. (2017). *RADNET: Radiologist Level Accuracy Using Deep Learning for HEMORRHAGE Detection in CT Scans*. http://arxiv.org/abs/1710.04934

24. Han, T., Nunes, V. X., De Freitas Souza, L. F., Marques, A. G., Silva, I. C. L., Junior, M. A. A. F., Sun, J., & Filho, P. P. R. (2020). Internet of Medical Things - Based on Deep Learning Techniques for Segmentation of Lung and Stroke Regions in CT Scans. *IEEE Access*, 8, 71117–71135. https://doi.org/10.1109/ACCESS.2020.2987932

25. Hssayeni, M. D., Croock, M. S., Salman, A. D., Al-Khafaji, H. F., Yahya, Z. A., & Ghoraani, B. (n.d.). *Intracranial Hemorrhage Segmentation Using a Deep Convolutional Model*. https://doi.org/10.13026/w8q8-ky94

26. Hu, X., Technologies, M., Luo, W., Hu, J., Guo, S., Huang, W., Scott, M. R., Wiest, R., & Reyes, M. (2020). *Brain SegNet: 3D Local Refinement Network for Brain Lesion Segmentation*. https://doi.org/10.21203/rs.2.14749/v3

27. Infogen Labs Inc., 2021.*Brain Stroke Detection Using Deep Learning*. https://www.linkedin.com/pulse/brain-stroke-detection-using-deep-learning-infogen-labs-

28. Jiang, L., Zhou, L., Yong, W., Cui, J., Geng, W., Chen, H., Zou, J., Chen, Y., Yin, X., & Chen, Y. C. (2021). A Deep Learning-Based Model for Prediction of Hemorrhagic Transformation After Stroke. *Brain Pathology*. https://doi.org/10.1111/bpa.13023

29. Jozwiak, R. Sobieszczuk, E., Ciszek, B., Wolski, P., Szklarski, M., & Domitrz, I. (2018). Preface. In *Advances in Intelligent Systems and Computing* (Vol. 647, pp. v–vii). Springer Verlag. https://doi.org/10.1007/978-3-319-66905-2

30. Kakkar, P., Kakkar, T., Patankar, T., & Saha, S. (2021). Current Approaches and Advances in the Imaging of Stroke. In *DMM Disease Models and Mechanisms* (Vol. 14, Issue 12). Company of Biologists Ltd. https://doi.org/10.1242/dmm.048785

31. Kamnitsas, K., Ledig, C., Newcombe, V. F. J., Simpson, J. P., Kane, A. D., Menon, D. K., Rueckert, D., & Glocker, B. (2017). Efficient Multi-scale 3D CNN with Fully Connected CRF for Accurate Brain Lesion Segmentation. *Medical Image Analysis*, 36, 61–78. https://doi.org/10.1016/j.media.2016.10.004

32. Karthik, R., Menaka, R., Hariharan, M., & Won, D. (2021). Ischemic Lesion Segmentation Using Ensemble of Multi-Scale Region Aligned CNN. *Computer Methods and Programs in Biomedicine*, 200. https://doi.org/10.1016/j.cmpb.2020.105831

33. Karthik, R., Menaka, R., Johnson, A., & Anand, S. (2020). Neuroimaging and Deep Learning for Brain Stroke Detection - A Review of Recent Advancements and Future Prospects. In *Computer Methods and Programs in Biomedicine* (Vol. 197). Elsevier Ireland Ltd. https://doi.org/10.1016/j.cmpb.2020.105728

34. Ker, J., Wang, L., Rao, J., & Lim, T. (2017). Deep Learning Applications in Medical Image Analysis. *IEEE Access*, 6, 9375–9379. https://doi.org/10.1109/ACCESS.2017.2788044

35. Kumar, M. A., Purohit, K. C., Gupta, A., Ghanshala, A., & Singh, A. (2022). Ischemic Stroke Prediction with B-LSTM Based on ECG Signals. *8th International Conference on Signal Processing and Communication (ICSC), Noida, India, 2022*, pp. 404–411. https://doi.org10.1109/ICSC56524.2022.10009499.

36. Lee, H., Lee, E.-J., Ham, S., Lee, H.-B., Lee, J. S., Kwon, S. U., Kim, J. S., Kim, N., Kang, D.-W., 2020. Machine Learning Approach to Identify Stroke within 4.5 Hours. *Stroke*, 51 (3), 860–866. https://doi.org/10.1161/STROKEAHA.119.027611.

37. Li, L., Wei, M., Liu, B., Atchaneeyasakul, K., Zhou, F., Pan, Z., Kumar, S. A., Zhang, J. Y., Pu, Y., Liebeskind, D. S., & Scalzo, F. (2021). Deep Learning for Hemorrhagic Lesion Detection and Segmentation on Brain CT Images. *IEEE Journal of Biomedical and Health Informatics*, 25(5), 1646–1659. https://doi.org/10.1109/JBHI.2020.3028243

38. Li, W., Li, Y., Qin, W., Liang, X., Xu, J., Xiong, J., & Xie, Y. (2020). Magnetic Resonance Image (MRI) Synthesis from Brain Computed Tomography (CT) Images Based on Deep Learning Methods for Magnetic Resonance (MR)-Guided Radiotherapy. *Quantitative Imaging in Medicine and Surgery*, 10(6), 1223–1236.

39. Liew, S. L., Anglin, J. M., Banks, N. W., Sondag, M., Ito, K. L., Kim, H., Chan, J., Ito, J., Jung, C., Khoshab, N., Lefebvre, S., Nakamura, W., Saldana, D., Schmiesing, A., Tran, C., Vo, D., Ard, T., Heydari, P., Kim, B., … Stroud, A. (2018). A Large, Open Source Dataset of Stroke Anatomical Brain Images and Manual Lesion Segmentations. *Scientific Data*, 5. https://doi.org/10.1038/sdata.2018.11

40. Liu, C.-F., Hsu, J., Xu, X., Ramachandran, S., Wang, V., Miller, M. I., Hillis, A. E., Faria, A. V., Wintermark, M., Warach, S. J., Albers, G. W., Davis, S. M., Grotta, J. C., Hacke, W., Kang, D.-W., Kidwell, C., Koroshetz, W. J., Lees, K. R., Lev, M. H., … Luby, M. (2021). Deep Learning-Based Detection and Segmentation of Diffusion Abnormalities in Acute Ischemic Stroke. *Communications Medicine*, 1(1), 61. https://doi.org/10.1038/s43856-021-00062-8

41. Lundervold, A. S., & Lundervold, A. (2019). An Overview of Deep Learning in Medical Imaging Focusing on MRI. In *Zeitschrift fur Medizinische Physik* (Vol. 29, Issue 2, pp. 102–127). Elsevier GmbH. https://doi.org/10.1016/j.zemedi.2018.11.002

42. Marbun, J. T., & Andayani, U. (2018). Classification of Stroke Disease Using Convolutional Neural Network. *Journal of Physics: Conference Series*, 978(1). https://doi.org/10.1088/1742-6596/978/1/012092

43. Menon, B. K. (2020). Neuroimaging in Acute Stroke. *Continuum (Minneapolis, Minn.)*, 26(2), 287–309. https://doi.org/10.1212/CON.0000000000000839

44. Menon, B. K., Campbell, B. C., Levi, C., & Goyal, M. (2015). Role of Imaging in Current Acute Ischemic Stroke Workflow for Endovascular Therapy. *Stroke*, 46(6), 1453–1461. https://doi.org/10.1161/STROKEAHA.115.009160

45. Nazari-Farsani, S., Yu, Y., Armindo, R. D., Lansberg, M., Liebeskind, D. S., Albers, G., Christensen, S., Levin, C. S., & Zaharchuk, G. (2023). Predicting Final Ischemic Stroke Lesions from Initial Diffusion-Weighted Images Using a Deep Neural Network. *NeuroImage: Clinical*, 37. https://doi.org/10.1016/j.nicl.2022.103278

46. Nie. (2016). *Estimating CT Image from MRI Data Using 3D Fully Convolutional Networks* (G. Carneiro, D. Mateus, L. Peter, A. Bradley, J. M. R. S. Tavares, V. Belagiannis, J. P. Papa, J. C. Nascimento, M. Loog, Z. Lu, J. S. Cardoso, & J. Cornebise, Eds.; Vol. 10008). Springer International Publishing. https://doi.org/10.1007/978-3-319-46976-8

47. Nie. (2017). *Medical Image Synthesis with Context-Aware Generative Adversarial Networks* (M. Descoteaux, L. Maier-Hein, A. Franz, P. Jannin, D. L. Collins, & S. Duchesne, Eds.; Vol. 10435). Springer International Publishing. https://doi.org/10.1007/978-3-319-66179-7

48. Nielsen, A., Hansen, M. B., Tietze, A., & Mouridsen, K. (2018). Prediction of Tissue Outcome and Assessment of Treatment Effect in Acute Ischemic Stroke Using Deep Learning. *Stroke*, 49(6), 1394–1401. https://doi.org/10.1161/STROKEAHA.117.019740

49. Nishi, H., Oishi, N., Ishii, A., Ono, I., Ogura, T., Sunohara, T., Chihara, H., Fukumitsu, R., Okawa, M., Yamana, N., Imamura, H., Sadamasa, N., Hatano, T., Nakahara, I., Sakai, N., & Miyamoto, S. (2020). Deep Learning-Derived High-Level Neuroimaging Features Predict Clinical Outcomes for Large Vessel Occlusion. *Stroke*, 1484–1492. https://doi.org/10.1161/STROKEAHA.119.028101

50. Nishio, M., Koyasu, S., Noguchi, S., Kiguchi, T., Nakatsu, K., Akasaka, T., Yamada, H., & Itoh, K. (2020). Automatic Detection of Acute Ischemic Stroke Using Non-contrast Computed Tomography and Two-Stage Deep Learning Model. *Computer Methods and Programs in Biomedicine*, 196. https://doi.org/10.1016/j.cmpb.2020.105711

51. Nogueira, R. G., Jadhav, A. P., Haussen, D. C., et al. (2018). Thrombectomy 6 to 24 Hours after Stroke with a Mismatch Between Deficit and Infarct. *The New England Journal of Medicine*, 378(1), 11–21.

52. Nugroho, A. K., Nugraheni, D. M. K., Putranto, T. A., Purnama, I. K. E. & Purnomo, M. H. (2022). Classification of Ischemic Stroke with Convolutional Neural Network (CNN) approach on b-1000 Diffusion-Weighted (DW) MRI. *EMITTER International Journal of Engineering Technology*, 195–216. https://doi.org/10.24003/emitter.v10i1.694

53. Ojha, N., & Banerji, S. (2022). Intracranial Hemorrhage Detection and Classification Using Deep Learning. *Augmenting Neurological Disorder Prediction and Rehabilitation Using Artificial Intelligence*, 1–14. https://doi.org/10.1016/B978-0-323-90037-9.00009-6

54. Park, S., Han, M.-K., & Hong, J.-H. (2021). *Deep Learning for Prediction of Mechanism in Acute Ischemic Stroke Using Brain MRI*. https://doi.org/10.21203/rs.3.rs-604141/v1

55. Patil, S., Rossi, R., Jabrah, D., & Doyle, K. (2022, June 24). Detection, Diagnosis and Treatment of Acute Ischemic Stroke: Current and Future Perspectives. *Frontiers in Medical Technology*, 4. https://doi.org/10.3389/fmedt.2022.748949

56. Potter, C. A., Vagal, A. S., Goyal, M., Nunez, D. B., Leslie-Mazwi, T. M., & Lev, M. H. (2019, October). CT for Treatment Selection in Acute Ischemic Stroke: A Code Stroke Primer. *RadioGraphics*, 39(6), 1717–1738. https://doi.org/10.1148/rg.2019190142

57. Puttagunta, M., & Ravi, S. (2021). Medical Image Analysis Based on Deep Learning Approach. *Multimedia Tools and Applications*, 80(16), 24365–24398. https://doi.org/10.1007/s11042-021-10707-4

58. Rokem, A. (2021). Detect-ing Brain Anomalies with Autoencoders. *Nature Computational Science*, 1, 569–570 (2021). https://www.nature.com/articles/s43588-021-00128-6#citeas

59. Shafaat, O. & Sotoudeh, H. (2023) Stroke Imaging. [Updated 2022 May 8]. In: *StatPearls [Internet]*. Treasure Island, FL: StatPearls Publishing;

60. Soun, J. E., Chow, D. S., Nagamine, M., Takhtawala, R. S., Filippi, C. G., Yu, W., & Chang, P. D. (2021). Artificial Intelligence and Acute Stroke Imaging. In *American Journal of Neuroradiology* (Vol. 42, Issue 1, pp. 2–11). American Society of Neuroradiology. https://doi.org/10.3174/ajnr.A6883

61. Soun, J., Chow, D., Nagamine, M., Takhtawala, R., Filippi, C., Yu, W., & Chang, P. (2020, November 26). Artificial Intelligence and Acute Stroke Imaging. *American Journal of Neuroradiology*, 42(1), 2–11. https://doi.org/10.3174/ajnr.a6883

62. Tang, Z. R., C. Y., H. R., & W. H. (2022). Predicting Hematoma Expansion in Intracerebral Hemorrhage from Brain CT Scans via K-nearest Neighbors Matting and Deep Residual Network. *Biomedical Signal Processing and Control*, 76, 103656.

63. Thiyagarajan, S. K. & Murugan, K. A. ((2021)) Systematic Review on Techniques Adapted for Segmentation and Classification of Ischemic Stroke Lesions from Brain MR Images. *Wireless Personal Communications*, 118, 1225–1244. https://doi.org/10.1007/s11277-021-08069-z

64. Tulay, E. E., Metin, B., Tarhan, N., & Arıkan, M. K. (2019). Multimodal Neuroimaging: Basic Concepts and Classification of Neuropsychiatric Diseases. In *Clinical EEG and Neuroscience* (Vol. 50, Issue 1, pp. 20–33). SAGE Publications Inc. https://doi.org/10.1177/1550059418782093

65. Types of Stroke | Johns Hopkins Medicine. (n.d.). Retrieved October 7, 2022, from https://www.hopkinsmedicine.org/health/conditions-and-diseases/stroke/types-of-stroke

66. Types of Stroke: Ischemic, Hemorrhagic, and TIA. (2022, August 23). WebMD. https://www.webmd.com/stroke/guide/types-stroke

67. Wajngarten, M., & Sampaio Silva, G. (2019). Hypertension and Stroke: Update on Treatment. *European Cardiology Review*, 14(2), 111–115. https://doi.org/10.15420/ECR.2019.11.1

68. Wang, X., Shen, T., Yang, S., Lan, J., Xu, Y., Wang, M., Zhang, J., & Han, X. (2021). A Deep Learning Algorithm for Automatic Detection and Classification of Acute Intracranial Hemorrhages in Head CT Scans. *NeuroImage: Clinical*, 32. https://doi.org/10.1016/j.nicl.2021.102785

69. Winder, A. J., Wilms, M., Amador, K., Flottmann, F., Fiehler, J., & Forkert, N. D. (2022). Predicting the Tissue Outcome of Acute Ischemic Stroke from Acute 4D Computed Tomography Perfusion Imaging Using Temporal Features and Deep Learning. *Frontiers in Neuroscience*, 16. https://doi.org/10.3389/fnins.2022.1009654

70. Woo, I., Lee, A., Jung, S. C., Lee, H., Kim, N., Cho, S. J., Kim, D., Lee, J., Sunwoo, L., & Kang, D. W. (2019). Fully Automatic Segmentation of Acute Ischemic Lesions on Diffusion-Weighted Imaging Using Convolutional Neural Networks: Comparison with Conventional Algorithms. *Korean Journal of Radiology*, 20(8), 1275–1284. https://doi.org/10.3348/kjr.2018.0615

71. Wu, W., Lu, Y., Mane, R. & Guan, C. (2020). Deep Learning for Neuroimaging Segmentation with a Novel Data Augmentation Strategy. *42nd Annual International Conference of the IEEE Engineering in Medicine & Biology Society (EMBC)*, Montreal, QC, Canada, 2020, pp. 1516–1519. https://doi.org/10.1109/EMBC44109.2020.9176537.

72. Xue, Y., Farhat, F. G., Boukrina, O., Barrett, A. M., Binder, J. R., Roshan, U. W., & Graves, W. W. (2020). A Multi-path 2.5 Dimensional Convolutional Neural Network System for Segmenting Stroke Lesions in Brain MRI Images. *NeuroImage: Clinical*, 25. https://doi.org/10.1016/j.nicl.2019.102118

73. Yalcn, S., & V. H. (2022). Brain Stroke Classification and Segmentation Using Encoder-Decoder Based Deep Convolutional Neural Networks. *Elsevier*. https://www.sciencedirect.com/science/article/abs/pii/S001048252200676X

74. Yan, W., Qu, G., Hu, W., Abrol, A., Cai, B., Qiao, C., Plis, S. M., Wang, Y. P., Sui, J., & Calhoun, V. D. (2022). Deep Learning in Neuroimaging: Promises and Challenges. *IEEE Signal Processing Magazine*, 39(2), 87–98. https://doi.org/10.1109/MSP.2021.3128348

75. Ye, H., Gao, F., Yin, Y., Guo, D., Zhao, P., Lu, Y., Wang, X., Bai, J., Cao, K., Song, Q., Zhang, H., Chen, W., Guo, X., & Xia, J. (2019). Precise Diagnosis of Intracranial Hemorrhage and Subtypes Using a Three-Dimensional Joint Convolutional and Recurrent Neural Network. *European Radiology*, 29(11), 6191–6201. https://doi.org/10.1007/s00330-019-06163-2

76. Yedavalli, V. S., Tong, E., Martin, D., Yeom, K. W., & Forkert, N. D. (2021). Artificial Intelligence in Stroke Imaging: Current and Future Perspectives. In *Clinical Imaging* (Vol. 69, pp. 246–254). Elsevier Inc. https://doi.org/10.1016/j.clinimag.2020.09.005

77. You, J., Tsang, A. C. O., Yu, P. L. H., Tsui, E. L. H., Woo, P. P. S., Lui, C. S. M., Leung, G. K. K. (2020, March) Automated Hierarchy Evaluation System of Large Vessel Occlusion in Acute Ischemia Stroke. *Frontiers in Neuroinformatics*, 14, 13. https://doi.org/10.3389/fninf.2020.00013. PMID: 32265682; PMCID: PMC7107673.

78. You, J., Yu, P. L., Tsang, A. C., Tsui, E. L., Woo, P. P., & Leung, G. K. (2019, June 18). Automated Computer Evaluation of Acute Ischemic Stroke and Large Vessel Occlusion. *arXiv Vanity*. https://www.arxiv-vanity.com/papers/1906.08059/

79. Yousef, R., Gupta, G., Yousef, N., & Khari, M. (2022). A Holistic Overview of Deep Learning Approach in Medical Imaging. *Multimedia Systems*, 28(3), 881–914. https://doi.org/10.1007/s00530-021-00884-5

80. Yu, J., Park, S., Kwon, S. H., Cho, K. H., & Lee, H. (2022). AI-Based Stroke Disease Prediction System Using ECG and PPG Bio-Signals. *IEEE Access*, 10, 43623–43638. https://doi.org/10.1109/ACCESS.2022.3169284

81. Yu, J., Park, S., Kwon, S. H., Ho, C. M. B., Pyo, C. S., & Lee, H. (2020). AI-Based Stroke Disease Prediction System Using Real-Time Electromyography Signals. *Applied Sciences (Switzerland)*, 10(19). https://doi.org/10.3390/app10196791

82. Yu, Y., Xie, Y., Thamm, T., Gong, E., Ouyang, J., Christensen, S., Marks, M. P., Lansberg, M. G., Albers, G. W., & Zaharchuk, G. (2021). Tissue at Risk and Ischemic Core Estimation Using Deep Learning in Acute Stroke. *American Journal of Neuroradiology*, 42(6), 1030–1037. https://doi.org/10.3174/ajnr.A7081

83. Zhang, Y., Liu, S., Li, C., & Wang, J. (2022). Application of Deep Learning Method on Ischemic Stroke Lesion Segmentation. In *Journal of Shanghai Jiaotong University (Science)* (Vol. 27, Issue 1, pp. 99–111). Shanghai Jiaotong University. https://doi.org/10.1007/s12204-021-2273-9

CHAPTER 2

Artificial Intelligence in Stroke Imaging

Lazzaro di Biase, Adriano Bonura, Pasquale Maria Pecoraro, Maria Letizia Caminiti, and Vincenzo Di Lazzaro

2.1 INTRODUCTION

"Time is brain" well summarizes in a single sentence what is the leading factor for clinical outcome in acute stroke: time. Indeed, every single minute after stroke onset, about 1.9 million neurons are lost resulting in an accelerated brain ageing of 3.6 years each hour without treatment.[1,2] Stroke is the second leading cause of death and the leading cause of disability all over the world.[3] Clinical significance of this disease has a huge economic impact, leading to healthcare expenditures of about USD 45.5 billion in the US and EUR 60 billion in Europe in 2017,[4] which corresponds to about 1.7% of healthcare spending.[5] Stroke can be haemorrhagic (13%) or ischemic (87%).[4] The latter is caused by cerebral hypoperfusion due to occlusion or subocclusion of a cerebral artery. Arterial revascularization is the only therapeutic option that can alter prognosis and functional outcomes, which can be performed by systemic thrombolysis with recombinant tissue factor (rtPA) and/or mechanical endothrombectomy.[6-9]

As mentioned above, the timing of these interventions is crucial, and it is closely associated with favourable outcomes.[2] The latest guidelines define an intervention time of up to 9 h for thrombolysis and up to 24 h for mechanical thrombectomy.[6-9]

Although innovative stroke diagnostic techniques, which will allow a more rapid diagnostic process, are still under evaluation,[10] classic neuroimaging techniques like CT and magnetic resonance imaging (MRI) play a key role in choosing the best therapeutic approach. In detail, brain CT (computed tomography) is fundamental in the acute phase to exclude the presence of haemorrhage, the main contraindication to performing revascularization therapy.[6-9] On the other hand, the use of iodinated contrast medium and CT angiography (CTA) allows to define the presence of occlusion of intracerebral main arterial

DOI: 10.1201/9781003264767-2

vessels, which is a condition needed for mechanical thrombectomy administration.[8,9] Instead, MRI allows a better definition of the diagnostic picture due to greater sensitivity and specificity compared with CT.[11] MRI is able to identify cerebral ischemia within the very first moments after the onset of symptoms (brain CT becomes positive after around 24 hours).

Artificial intelligence (AI) algorithms have been proposed to solve several issues in the neurology field in order to improve the diagnosis, symptoms monitoring, or therapy management of diseases like Parkinson's disease,[12–16] dystonia,[17,18] or epilepsy,[19,20] and an emerging field is stroke in which the impact in terms of disability spared and mortality lowered is even higher.

Use of AI for recognition and processing of neuroimaging data is a hot research topic in the last few years (Figure 2.4). With the Rapid.AI software,[21] the new American and European stroke guidelines have already incorporated the use of AI systems into clinical practice.[6–9] This chapter will review the various neuroimaging-based AI systems used in stroke and evaluate their diagnostic performance. The different software have been classified into primary prevention, diagnosis, and prognosis software.

2.2 STROKE PREVENTION AI SYSTEMS

Stroke prevention is based on risk factors recognition and treatment.[22] Most common aetiologies are cardioembolic and atherosclerotic strokes.[4] For the latter, it is important to assess the presence of hypertension, dyslipidemia, and diabetes mellitus, which may predispose to the formation and growth of atherosclerotic plaques. Such vessel alterations may lead to vessel occlusion or rupture resulting in embolization of thrombus. Early recognition of alteration of neck and intracranial arterial vessels and administration of appropriate therapies results in a reduction of ischemic risk.[22] Neural networks can assist physicians in neck lesion recognition. A technique to identify atherosclerosis of carotid arteries based on machine learning (ML) recognition of white matter lesions detected by MRI was tested on 401 subjects (190 patients with carotid stenosis, 211 healthy subjects). White matter lesions can have different aetiologies; they can be due to transient hypoafflux from arterial stenosis, small vessel alterations, genetic disease, or inflammatory diseases such as multiple sclerosis.[23] A computational approach in the above study was implemented through support vector machine (SVM). Results showed an accuracy rate of 97.5% with a sensitivity of 96.4% and specificity of 97.9% in discerning between white matter lesion due to carotid stenosis, multiple sclerosis, small vessel disease and healthy subjects.[24]

Doppler ultrasonography is the most rapid and inexpensive method for evaluation of carotid arteries, which provides structural and dynamic information on blood vessels and flow. In particular, myointimal thickness is a marker of cardiovascular risk. Both stroke and myocardial infarction risk increase with carotid myointimal thickness. The odds ratio per standard deviation increase (0.163 mm) was 1.41 for stroke and 1.43 for myocardial infarction.[25] A method to automatically calculate carotid artery myointimal thickness was proposed using deep learning (DL) and ML on ultrasound images; 396 b-mode ultrasound images of the common carotid artery from 203 patients were used. Results show that 88% of patients with increased myointimal thickness (cut off 0.9 mm) were correctly recognized by AI. This software demonstrated greater accuracy than market software.[26] In another study statistical pattern recognition was used to measure myointimal thickness from ultrasound images of the internal carotid artery. The algorithm was tested on 55 longitudinal ultrasound images by comparing them with manual segmentation. Results showed a correlation coefficient between automatic and manual measurement of 93.3% with a slight underestimation of Intima-Media Thickness (IMT) by the automatic method.[27] Another study used morphometric analysis to differentiate an atherosclerotic intra-carotid plaque from a floating intraluminal thrombus based on CT vascular images. The model demonstrated a sensitivity of 87.5% and a specificity of 71.4% with a ranged accuracy from 65.2% to 76.4%.[28]

2.3 STROKE DIAGNOSIS AI SYSTEMS

Stroke is an acute onset disease in which timing of intervention is the main factor that can change a patient's outcome.[2] Revascularization therapies cannot be separated from imaging examinations such as brain CT and CT angio. Noncontrast brain CT allows to exclude intracranial haemorrhage, which is one of the main contraindications to revascularization therapies.[6–8] CT imaging provides automatic recognition and discrimination between healthy subjects; ischemic and haemorrhagic lesions is the topic of several studies. For example, possibility of using structural co-occurrence matrix (SCM) to differentiate ischemic from haemorrhagic strokes on CT images was evaluated, achieving specificity of 99.1%, sensitivity of 97%, and with an F score of 98% and accuracy of 98%.[29] Another method used analysis of brain tissue density (ABTD) for the differential diagnosis between healthy subjects and ischemic or haemorrhagic tissue with a diagnostic accuracy of 99.30%.[30]

In the first few hours, CT rarely shows the presence of an ischemic lesion that is identified with a hypodensity compared with healthy tissue. However, in some cases, especially when the lesion is very extensive, cytotoxic oedema and thus hypodensity may be present. The extent of ischemic injury correlates with haemorrhagic risk post revascularization procedures, so it is common to quantify the extent of hypodensity as an indication for performing thrombolysis and/or thrombectomy.[6–8] ASPECTS (Alberta Stroke Program Early CT Score)[31] allows a score from 1 to 10 to be assigned to the extent of ischemic lesions in the anterior circulation territory, and, based on this, a decision can be made on whether or not to perform revascularization therapies.[6–8] iSchemaView and Brainomix have implemented AIs in their software with the ability to recognize hypodensities on CT and automatically calculate ASPECTS. ASPECT by iSchemaView[32] is based on random forest learning (RFL) technology that compares images from both sides of the brain by returning a numerical ASPECTS value. A study of 152 cases was performed comparing the diagnostic accuracy in terms of consensus score in calculating ASPECTS between AI and 2 neuroradiologists. Automated ASPECTS showed significantly better performance than its human counterpart (kappa human consensus 57% vs. 90%).[32] E-ASPECT by Brainomix

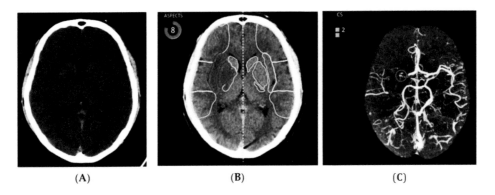

FIGURE 2.1   (a) Brain CT shows ischemic lesions in the territory of the right middle cerebral artery at the level of the insula and basal ganglia and (b) ischemic lesions of the same patient detected by e-ASPECT (ASPECTS = 8). (c) Automatic detection of right middle cerebral artery occlusion by e-CTA. Collateral score = 2. (Reproduced under the terms and conditions of the Creative Commons Attribution (CC BY) licence from Zelenak et al.)[68]

has been evaluated by several studies[33–37] (Figure 2.1a and 2.1b). Seker et al.[33] showed better diagnostic performance of the automated system in calculating ASPECTS compared with four neuroradiologists with kappa of 92% vs. 75%, respectively.[33] In another study, the ASPECTS calculated by AI and a neuroradiologist were compared with blood flow and perfusion assessed by CT perfusion.[34] Software results were similar to neuroradiologist's ones and showed a high degree of correlation with cerebral blood flow (CBV).[34] In several studies e-ASPECT showed better performance than neuroradiologists,[35–37] and reduced scoring time by 34%.[35]

New acute stroke management guidelines have expanded the time window for performing thrombolysis to 9 hours and for thrombectomy to 24 hours.[6–8] Choice of administration of revascularization therapies depends on the relationship between ischemic core and ischemic penumbra. The ischemic core represents the portion of brain tissue that is not perfused and therefore not recoverable. Penumbra, on the other hand, represents a portion of the brain around the core that is hypoperfused but potentially recoverable if flow restoration occurs. The greater the ratio between these two portions, the greater the chance of recovery of function if therapeutic procedures are performed. Evaluation can be implemented by study with brain perfusion CT or MRI with PWI (perfusion-weighted imaging) sequences. Development of software trained in the recognition of cerebral perfusion imaging made it possible to extend the therapeutic windows, increasing the number of patients treated and functional recovery. The most widely used software currently is RAPIDAI by iSchemaView[38] (Figure 2.2). It was validated in the DEFUSE 2[39] and DEFUSE 3[40] study and has received FDA approval (2013) and Conformité Européenne marking in Europe. RAPIDAI[21] can analyse CT and MRI perfusion images and return as output colorimetric maps indicating ischemic core and ischemic penumbra.

On CT, RAPIDAI is able to measure the attenuation of the height curves of each pixel in the arterial and venous phases since the arrival of the contrast fluid. A mathematical model –

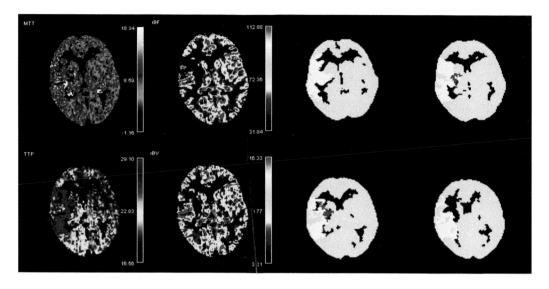

FIGURE 2.2   (a) Perfusion maps showing penumbra in territory of right middle cerebral artery and (b) relative mismatch of 95.8%. (RAPID software). (Reproduced under the terms and conditions of the Creative Commons Attribution (CC BY) licence from Zelenak et al.)[68]

circular deconvolution – is used to estimate contrast concentration in vessels based on attenuation. Information are used to calculate cerebral blood volume (CBV), mean transit time (MTT), time to peak concentration (T-max), and cerebral flow for each pixel. A perfusion map is generated based on these data.[21] Accuracy for ischemic core prediction was 83%.[40,41] For MRI RAPIDAI co-registers DWI (diffusion-weighted imaging) and PWI data and then evaluates hypoperfused areas and areas with vasogenic oedema by calculating volumetric mismatch ratio and converting informations into perfusion maps. Sensibility of RAPID MRI is 100%, and specificity is 91%.[40,41]

RAPID technology has been used in large stroke trials: EXTEND-IA,[42] SWIFT PRIME,[43] CRISP,[44] DEFUSE 2[39] and 3,[40] eDAWN[45].

iSchemaView has also developed software for recognition of large vessel occlusion (LVO) by angioTC.

Viz.ai is a 2018 FDA-approved software for LVO stroke recognition in CT images (Viz LVO) and CT perfusion (Viz CTP) images. Viz LVO can recognize presence LVO. An analysis of 650 patients showed a sensitivity of 82%, specificity of 94%, PPV (positive predictive value) of 77%, and NPV (negative predictive value) of 95%.[46] Another study conducted on 610 patients showed an accuracy of 87.9%.[47] Once the pattern is recognized, it sends an alert to the stroke team, via mobile phone application, also ensuring a reduction in intervention time.[46] Viz CTP, on the other hand, can recognize alterations in perfusion; it also has a motion correction system.

Brainomix: StrokeSuite guarantees a software series that can recognize LVO (e-CTA) (Figure 2.1c), calculate ASPECT (e-ASPECT), and give perfusion maps in CT and MRI (Olea Sphere- e-CTP) (Figure 2.3). e-CTA received CE marking in 2018. Thanks to

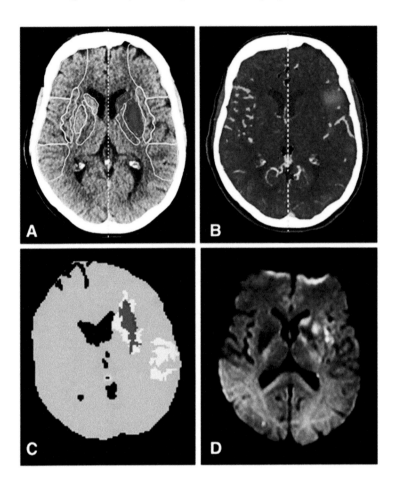

FIGURE 2.3   Clinical case of ischemic stroke from left M1 occlusion with NIHSS:17. E-ASPECTS (a) is 8 with involvement of the caudate head and nucleus lentiformis, collateral e-CTA score was 2 (54%, b), and hypoperfused area (c) is significantly smaller, so it performed thrombectomy with complete recanalization (mTICI 3) and NIHSS: 0.36 hours follow-up MRI (d) shows incomplete infarction of the striated area only. (Reproduced under the terms and conditions of the Creative Commons Attribution (CC BY) licence from Mokli et al.)[69]

convolutional neural networks (CNNs) it can detect structure occlusions in one to two minutes. Also, it allows to evaluate collateral circles such as RAPIDAI and to discriminate left-right asymmetry. It gives heat maps and also provides vessel density percentage scores. The Grunwald et al. study conducted on 98 patients assessed e-CTA performance against three experienced neuroradiologists. Consensus score was 90%, and sensitivity and specificity were 99% and 94%.[48] In another study, both e-ASPECT and e-CTA and results obtained on ASPECTS and collateral circles correlated with the mRS (modified Rankin scale) at three months.[49]

e-CTP (formerly Olea Sphere) can show CT and MR perfusion maps, volume and ratio mismatch assessment, and DWI maps. Images can be shared via picture archiving and

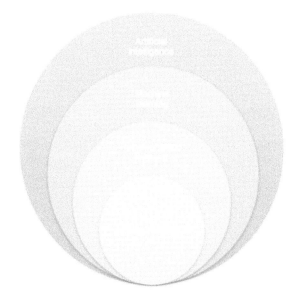

b

Machine learning algorithms and models	Sup L	Unsup L	Reinf L	Rep L	DL
linear regression	•				
logistic regression	•				
support vector machines (SVM)	•				
decision trees	•				
random forest	•				
naïve bayes	•				
k-nearest neighbours algorithm (k-NN)	•				
similarity learning	•				
k-means clustering		•			
probabilistic clustering		•			
mixture models (e.g. Gaussian mixture)		•			
association rule		•			
hidden Markov model		•			
hierarchical clustering		•			
linear discriminant analysis (LDA)	•	•			
principal component analysis (PCA)		•			
singular-value decomposition (SVD)		•			
Q-learning			•		
learning automaton			•		
temporal difference			•		
state-action-reward-state-action (SARSA)			•		
autoencoder		•		•	•
shallow neural networks (one layer)	•	•		•	
deep neural networks			•	•	•

FIGURE 2.4 (a) Deep learning is a type of representation learning, which is a type of ML, which is a subfield of AI. (b) A summary representation of the most common ML algorithms and models. Sup L: supervised learning: labelled data are used. Unsup L: unsupervised learning: unlabelled data is used. Semi-supervised learning: a mixture of supervised and unsupervised learning. Reinf L: reinforcement learning: learning through action (rewarding the right actions and punishing the wrong ones). Rep L: learning by representation: automatic feature generation. DL: deep learning: hierarchical representation learning. (Reproduced under the terms and conditions of the Creative Commons Attribution (CC BY) licence from Mokli et al.)[69]

communication system (PACS) and sent via email. In one study, 487 angiographies were evaluated; the sensitivity was 84% and specificity 96%.[50]

Another AI for perfusion and CT vascuolar image recognition is GE Healthcare Fast Stroke. Software also gives images on collateral circulation and it allows visualization of ischemic core and penumbra through a display called ColorViz. Such system highlights the three cerebral vascular phases (arterial, parenchymal, and venous) in a single map with different colours allowing assessment of altered cerebral perfusion and the presence of collateral circulations much faster than a three-phase CT angio study.[51]

CNN to identify ischemic lesions in MRI has been proposed. System was trained on the MRI dataset from the ISLES 2015 Challenge.[52] Each dataset includes four MRI sequences: T1, T2, FLAIR, and DWI. The results show a diagnostic accuracy level in recognizing ischemic lesions of about 70%.[53]

2.4 STROKE PROGNOSIS AI SYSTEMS

One of the major determinants of a worst prognosis is the presence of intracranial haemorrhage.[54] This complication may present ab initio, as a haemorrhagic stroke, or it may result from haemorrhagic transformation of an ischemic stroke.[54] Revascularization therapy has haemorrhagic infarction as its main side effect.[6-8] An AI capable of predicting haemorrhagic transformation of an ischemic stroke undergoing thrombolysis has been proposed based on CT images.[55] Clinical records and CT images of 116 patients were used to train the algorithm. An additional input was the patients' clinical features. Predictive performance reached an ROC AUC of 0.74.[55] In intracranial haemorrhage, however, the most important negative prognostic factor is hematoma expansion. One study used SVM to predict intracranial hematoma expansion in patients with spontaneous intracerebral haemorrhage (ICH).[56] A study evaluated CT images performed within 6 h after onset of ICH symptoms of 1,157 patients and follow-up performed within 72 h. The software showed a sensitivity of 81.3%, a specificity of 84.8%, an accuracy of 83.3%, and an ROC AUC of 89%.[56]

Other software has been used to predict good reperfusions post endovascular treatment. The DL-based algorithm was trained with CT vascular images of 1,301 patients extracted from the MR CLEAN registry. The model showed an ROC AUC of 0.71 for prediction of good clinical outcome and 0.65 for prediction of complete reperfusion.[57]

Ischemic lesions characteristics found in MRI were used to predict clinical outcomes. In one study, Hope et al. implemented an algorithm capable of making predictions of the severity of post-stroke cognitive impairment.[58] The inputs were a database with cognitive scores and encephalic MRI images. The system related lesions to imaging, demographic, and clinical information. Results showed an $R^2 = 0.84$.[58] In another study, voxel analysis on MRI images of stroke was used to predict long-term motor outcomes. The study showed an R of 0.83 and RMSE of 0.68.[59]

2.5 DISCUSSION

2.5.1 Clinical Impact

Use of AI systems in clinical stroke practice is still limited to a few examples. Table 2.1 summarizes the results of the most relevant studies focused on AI solutions for stroke

TABLE 2.1 Summary of reviewed paper on the use of AI in stroke

Study	AI	Imaging method	Aim	Sample	Results	Conclusion
24	SVM	MRI	Identification of ATR etiology of white matter lesion	401	Accuracy rate 97.5%, sensitivity 96.4%, 97.9%	AI showed good accuracy in the identification of white matter lesions
26	DL and ML	Ultrasonography	Calculation of CA thickness	203	Error on test set DL1 = 0.126 ± 0.134. 88% with increased MT correctly recognized	Low errors in carotid thickness values identification compared with human accuracy
27	PR	Ultrosonography	Calculation of CA thickness	55	Correlation coefficient 93.3%	High accuracy of carotid thickness values identifications compared with experts
28	ML	CTA	Differential between plaque and intrlauminal thrombus		Sensitivity 87.5%, specificity 71.4%, accuracy:65.2-76.4%	AI is able to differentiate between a atherosclerotic plaque and intraluminal thrombus
29	SCM	CT	Differential between hemorrhagic and ischemic stroke		Specificity = 99.1% Sensitivity = 97% FScore = 98% ACC = 98%	AI shows high accuracy in differentiate between ischemia and hemorrhage
30	ABTD	CT	Differential between hemorrhagic and ischemic stroke		Diagnostic accuracy: 99.3%	AI shows high accuracy in differentiate between ischemia and hemorrhage
32	RFL – ASPECT (iSchemaView)	CT	Calculation of ASPECT (AI vs. neuroradiologists)	152	kappa human consensus (57% vs. 90%)	AI show better accuracy in ASPECT calculation than radiologists
33	RFL-E-ASPECT(Brainomix)	CT	Calculation of ASPECT (AI vs. neuroradiologists)	43	kappa of 75% vs 92%,	AI show better accuracy in ASPECT calculation than radiologists
34	RFL-RAPID CTP/ E-ASPECT(Brainomix)	CTP	Calculation of ASPECT (AI and neuroradiologists) and association with CTP core	184		Software results were similar to neuroradiologists ones and showed a high degree of correlation with cerebral blood flow

(Continued)

TABLE 2.1 (*Continued*) Summary of reviewed paper on the use of AI in stroke

Study	AI	Imaging method	Aim	Sample	Results	Conclusion
35	RFL-E-ASPECT(Brainomix)	CT	Calculation of ASPECT (AI vs. neuroradiologists), baseline 24-36h	132	AI sensitivity ~45%, specificity ~92%, accuracy ~86%	AI doesn't show an inferiority with radiologists in ASPECT calculation
36	RFL-E-ASPECT(Brainomix)	CT	Calculation of ASPECT (AI vs. neuroradiologists) within 6 hours	119	AI sensitivity 83% vs human 73%, specificity 57% vs 84%	AI shows better sensitivity and lower specificity in ASPECT calculation compared with radiologists
37	RFL-E-ASPECT(Brainomix)	CT and MRi DWI	Calculation of ASPECT (AI vs. neuroradiologists) and correlation with MRi	34	AI sensitivity 46%, specificity 95%. AI correlation coefficient 0.44 vs humans 0.19–0.38	AI shows greater correlation with MR images than radiologists in calculating ASPECT
39	RFL-RAPID	MRI PWI	Thrombectomy within 12 h using RM PWI	138	RAPID MRI sensitivity 100%, specificity 91%	DEFUSE 2 trial
40	RFL-RAPID	CTP, RM PWI	Thrombectomy between 6-16h using CTP	182	RAPID CTP accuracy: 83%, RAPID MRI sensitivity 100%, specificity 91%	DEFUSE 3 trial
46	CNN-Viz.ai	CTA	Identification of LVOs from CTA images	650	Sensitivity 82%, specificity 94%, PPV 77%, NPV 95%	Viz.ai is able to detect LVOs with good accuracy
47	CNN-Viz.ai	CTA	Identification of LVOs from CTA images	610	Accuracy of 87.9%	Viz.ai is able to detect LVOs with good accuracy
48	CNN-eCTA (Brainomix)	CTA	Identification of LVOs from CTA images	98	Sensitivity: 99%, Specificity: 94%	AI is able to detect LVOs with high accuracy
49	CNN-eCTA + RFL-eASPECT	CT, CTA	Correlation between ischemic lesions, collateral circles and clinical outcome	102	Correlation rS = 0.322, 95%CI 0.131 to 0.482	Good correlation between functional outcome and eASPECT and eCTA values

No.	Method	Modality	Task	Sample	Results	Conclusion
50	CNN- eCTA	CTA	I Identification of LVOs from CTA images	487	Specificity = 96% Sensitivity = 84%	AI is able to detect LVOs with good accuracy
51	ColorViz (GE Healthcare)	CTA, CTP	Evaluation of collateral circulation compared with CTA	86	Accordance with CTA r = 0.735–0.839	Good accordance between radiologists using ColorViz and CTA images
53	CNN	MRI	Identify ischemic lesions	ISLES	Accuracy 70%	Average accuracy in automated identification of ischemic images.
55	SVM	CT	Prediction of thrombolysisi related hemorrhage	116	AUC = 0.744	Good accuracy in hemorrhage prediction after thrombolysis
56	SVM	CT	Prediction of intracranial hematoma expansion in ICH patients	1157	Sensitivity = 81.3% Specificity of 84.8% ACC = 83.3% AUC = 89%	Good accuracy in hematoma expansion prediction
57	DL	CTA	Prediction of good reperfusion after EVT	1301	AUC = 0.71 for good clinical outcome, AUC = 0.65 for prediction of complete reperfusion	Good accuracy in reperfusion rate prediction after thrombectomy
58	GPR	MRI	Prediction of speech skills using ischemic lesion characteristics	270	R^2 = 0.84	AI shows a correlation between ischemic lesion characteristics and speech outcome
59	GPR	MRI	Prediction upper limb motor function using ischemia characteristics	50	R = 0.83, RMSE = 0.68	AI shows correlation between ischemic lesions characteristic and upper motor function outcome

patients. Nevertheless, the impact in the clinic has been disruptive.[60] The main example is the use of RAPIDAI software for the identification of ischemic penumbra by CT perfusion. The use of such software in the DAWN,[45] DEFUSE 2[39] and 3[40], and EXTEND[61] trials, and the subsequent inclusion of extended windows in the new guidelines, has markedly changed the decision-making and treatment algorithms in the acute phase of stroke. While these trials have demonstrated a reduction in mortality and functional outcome in patients treated with revascularization therapies in the extended windows compared with patients treated with medical therapy,[40,45,61], this development and modification of decision-making algorithms has not been supported by a functional change in hospital protocols.[62] In fact, there has been an increase in the complexity of decision-making processes that has led to a slowdown in clinical decision-making and thus in inter-hospital transport and resource management.[62]

Although the other systems are still little used in clinical practice, the feature that needs to be mentioned is the high diagnostic accuracy of AI software, equal to or even higher than its human counterpart, both in the primary prevention phase and in the recognition of carotid vessel changes by ultrasonography[26,27,28] or white matter lesions by MRI,[24] as well as in the diagnostic phase. In addition to CT perfusion systems, which provide recognition of perfusion alterations that cannot be recognized by the human counterpart, ASPECTS calculation systems have been designed with better diagnostic accuracy than experienced neuroradiologists.[32,35–37] Even in the recognition of stroke from LVO by CTA, commercially available software allows one to achieve higher diagnostic accuracies than humans.[46,51]

Another advantage offered by these systems is the diagnostic timing. AI systems provide rapid diagnosis leading to a significant shortening of intervention time. In a strictly time-dependent condition such as stroke, this translates into faster therapies with reductions in mortality and improvement in functional outcomes. A RAPIDAI study showed a reduction of about 35 minutes in door to first pass time (treatment initiation) and 37 minutes in door to recanalization time.[63]

2.6 COST-EFFECTIVENESS OF AI FOR STROKE

Considering the net cost of AI solutions, around tens of thousands USD (e.g., RAPIDAI starts at USD 12,000), the estimated economic benefit is enormous. Estimated economic impact of AI for LVO recognition was analysed through the "health technology assessment method" (HTA), which allows us to assess the potential value of an early-stage technology.[64] Results showed a savings per patient of USD 156 and an incremental QALYs (quality adjusted life years) of +0.07%.[64] This translates into an annual savings of about 11 million USD (in UK).[64]

The real economic impact in healthcare of CT perfusion software and extended therapeutic windows has not yet been calculated. However, a cost-effectiveness estimate for thrombectomy was made following the DAWN (Clinical Mismatch in the Triage of Wake

Up and Late Presenting Strokes Undergoing Neurointervention With Trevo) and DEFUSE 3 (Endovascular Therapy Following Imaging Evaluation for Ischemic Stroke) criteria. Results show an increase in QALY by following the trials criteria, compared to not following the trials criteria.[65] At the same time, another study highlighted the potential benefits in using CT perfusion even outside the current guidelines. The question that arises is whether the use of AI in all cases of severe moderate stroke (i.e., that which can benefit from thrombectomy) may be unsustainable in terms of healthcare costs. Analysis conducted shows that while the use of CT perfusion in any stroke leads to an increase in healthcare cost per patient (1.19% per patient imaging cost, 33.25% per patient treatment costs), it results in an increase in patients treated with better functional outcomes, a reduction in patients with severe disability, and no change in mortality. These considerations lead to a reduction in QALY compared with the use of perfusion CT according to current guidelines, thus showing a five-year payback.[66]

2.6 LIMITATIONS OF AI USE IN STROKE PATIENTS

Fundamental in AI use in stroke imaging is the robustness of computer systems, that is, the ability to cope with execution errors. The greatest points of vulnerability in AI systems for stroke are the overfitting effect and the black-box effect.[67] Such accurate image recognition systems require huge amounts of data. Moreover, quality of this data is a fundamental requirement to prevent the model from learning to distinguish noise instead of signal. This circumstance, in systems with the machine learning (ML) model, leads to the problem of overfitting. Indeed, such systems tend to be extremely reliable in the training dataset, but such good performance is not replicable and generalizable in other datasets. The black-box effect, on the other hand, refers to the human difficulty in interpreting the learning algorithm. This problem leads to not recognizing the patterns and signals that the software is learning; this is a typical issue in DL models. To overcome this problem, many DL models have incorporated tools such as saliency maps.[67]

Such limitations are limiting the diffusion of these systems, as they do not allow the recognition of the behaviour of the computer system and the maintenance of high accuracy values over time. Therefore, it is essential to develop standardized methods for testing the performance of different models.

2.7 CONCLUSION

Exponential growth of AI system in stroke imaging will lead to more accurate, faster, and more sustainable assessment of stroke. However, such technological innovation in the clinical setting must be supported in a constant update of hospital protocols and proper management of intra-department transport and resources. This, together with continued physician education on new guidelines, would go a long way towards maximizing the reduction in endovascular stroke intervention time.

REFERENCES

1. Saver JL. Time is brain—Quantified. *Stroke.* 2006;37(1):263–266. doi:10.1161/01.STR. 0000196957.55928.ab

2. Risitano A, Toni D. Time is brain: Timing of revascularization of brain arteries in stroke. *Eur Heart J Suppl.* 2020;22(Supplement_L):L155–L159. doi:10.1093/eurheartj/suaa157

3. Katan M, Luft A. Global burden of stroke. *Semin Neurol.* 2018;38(02):208–211. doi:10.1055/s-0038-1649503

4. Virani SS, Alonso A, Aparicio HJ, et al. Heart disease and stroke statistics-2021 update: A report from the American heart association. *Circulation.* 2021;143(8):e254–e743. doi:10.1161/ CIR.0000000000000950

5. Luengo-Fernandez R, Violato M, Candio P, Leal J. Economic burden of stroke across Europe: A population-based cost analysis. *Eur Stroke J.* 2020;5(1):17–25. doi:10.1177/2396987319883160

6. Berge E, Whiteley W, Audebert H, et al. European Stroke Organisation (ESO) guidelines on intravenous thrombolysis for acute ischaemic stroke. *Eur Stroke J.* 2021;6(1):I–LXII. doi:10.1177/2396987321989865

7. Powers WJ, Rabinstein AA, Ackerson T, et al. Guidelines for the early management of patients with acute ischemic stroke: 2019 update to the 2018 guidelines for the early management of acute ischemic stroke: A guideline for healthcare professionals from the American heart association/American stroke association. *Stroke.* 2019;50(12):e344–e418. doi:10.1161/ STR.0000000000000211

8. Toni D, Mangiafico S, Agostoni E, et al. Intravenous thrombolysis and intra-arterial interventions in acute ischemic stroke: Italian Stroke Organisation (ISO)-SPREAD guidelines. *Int J Stroke Off J Int Stroke Soc.* 2015;10(7):1119–1129. doi:10.1111/ijs.12604

9. Turc G, Bhogal P, Fischer U, et al. European Stroke Organisation (ESO) - European Society for Minimally Invasive Neurological Therapy (ESMINT) guidelines on mechanical thrombectomy in acute ischemic stroke. *J Neurointerventional Surg.* Published online February 26, 2019: Neurintsurg-2018–014569. doi:10.1136/neurintsurg-2018–014569

10. di Biase L, Bonura A, Caminiti ML, Pecoraro PM, Di Lazzaro V. Neurophysiology tools to lower the stroke onset to treatment time during the golden hour: Microwaves, bioelectrical impedance and near infrared spectroscopy. *Ann Med.* 54(1):2658–2671. doi:10.1080/07853890. 2022.2124448

11. Chalela JA, Kidwell CS, Nentwich LM, et al. Magnetic resonance imaging and computed tomography in emergency assessment of patients with suspected acute stroke: A prospective comparison. *Lancet Lond Engl.* 2007;369(9558):293–298. doi:10.1016/S0140–6736(07)60151-2

12. di Biase L, Di Santo A, Caminiti ML, et al. Gait analysis in Parkinson's disease: An overview of the most accurate markers for diagnosis and symptoms monitoring. *Sensors.* 2020;20(12):E3529. doi:10.3390/s20123529

13. di Biase L, Tinkhauser G, Martin Moraud E, Caminiti ML, Pecoraro PM, Di Lazzaro V. Adaptive, personalized closed-loop therapy for Parkinson's disease: Biochemical, neurophysiological, and wearable sensing systems. *Expert Rev Neurother.* 2021;21(12):1371–1388. doi:10. 1080/14737175.2021.2000392

14. d'Angelis O, Di Biase L, Vollero L, Merone M. IoT architecture for continuous long term monitoring: Parkinson's disease case study. *Internet Things.* 2022;20:100614. doi:10.1016/j. iot.2022.100614

15. di Biase L, Raiano L, Caminiti ML, Pecoraro PM, Lazzaroo VD. 3- Artificial intelligence in Parkinson's disease—Symptoms identification and monitoring. In: Pillai AS, Menon B, eds. *Augmenting Neurological Disorder Prediction and Rehabilitation Using Artificial Intelligence.* Academic Press; 2022:35–52. doi:10.1016/B978-0-323-90037-9.00003–5

16. Pillai AS, Menon B, eds. Augmenting neurological disorder prediction and rehabilitation using artificial intelligence. In: *Augmenting Neurological Disorder Prediction and Rehabilitation Using Artificial Intelligence.* Academic Press; 2022:i–iii. doi:10.1016/B978-0-323-90037-9.00022-9

17. di Biase L, Di Santo A, Caminiti ML, Pecoraro PM, Di Lazzaro V. Classification of dystonia. *Life.* 2022;12(2):206. doi:10.3390/life12020206

18. di Biase L, Di Santo A, Caminiti ML, Pecoraro PM, Carbone SP, Di Lazzaro V. Dystonia diagnosis: Clinical neurophysiology and genetics. *J Clin Med.* 2022;11(14):4184. doi:10.3390/jcm11144184

19. Kaur T, Diwakar A, Kirandeep null, et al. Artificial intelligence in epilepsy. *Neurol India.* 2021;69(3):560–566. doi:10.4103/0028–3886.317233

20. Artificial intelligence and computational approaches for epilepsy – PMC. Accessed October 26, 2022. https://www.ncbi.nlm.nih.gov/pmc/articles/PMC7494883/

21. http://fyra.io. RAPID Automated CT Perfusion in Clinical Practice. *Practical Neurology.* Accessed July 15, 2022. https://practicalneurology.com/articles/2019-nov-dec/rapid-automated-ct-perfusion-in-clinical-practice

22. Kleindorfer DO, Towfighi A, Chaturvedi S, et al. 2021 Guideline for the prevention of stroke in patients with stroke and transient ischemic attack: A guideline From the American Heart Association/American Stroke Association. *Stroke.* 2021;52(7):e364–e467. doi:10.1161/STR.0000000000000375

23. Leite M, Rittner L, Appenzeller S, Ruocco HH, Lotufo R. Etiology-based classification of brain white matter hyperintensity on magnetic resonance imaging. *J Med Imaging.* 2015;2(1):014002. doi:10.1117/1.JMI.2.1.014002

24. Bento M, Souza R, Salluzzi M, Rittner L, Zhang Y, Frayne R. Automatic identification of atherosclerosis subjects in a heterogeneous MR brain imaging data set. *Magn Reson Imaging.* 2019;62:18–27. doi:10.1016/j.mri.2019.06.007

25. Bots ML, Hoes AW, Koudstaal PJ, Hofman A, Grobbee DE. Common carotid intima-media thickness and risk of stroke and myocardial infarction. *Circulation.* 1997;96(5):1432–1437. doi:10.1161/01.CIR.96.5.1432

26. Biswas M, Kuppili V, Araki T, et al. Deep learning strategy for accurate carotid intima-media thickness measurement: An ultrasound study on Japanese diabetic cohort. *Comput Biol Med.* 2018;98:100–117. doi:10.1016/j.compbiomed.2018.05.014

27. Menchón-Lara RM, Sancho-Gómez JL. Fully automatic segmentation of ultrasound common carotid artery images based on machine learning. *Neurocomputing.* 2015;151:161–167. doi:10.1016/j.neucom.2014.09.066

28. Thornhill RE, Lum C, Jaberi A, et al. Can shape analysis differentiate free-floating internal carotid artery thrombus from atherosclerotic plaque in patients evaluated with CTA for stroke or transient ischemic attack? *Acad Radiol.* 2014;21(3):345–354. doi:10.1016/j.acra.2013.11.011

29. Peixoto SA, Rebouças Filho PP. Neurologist-level classification of stroke using a Structural Co-Occurrence Matrix based on the frequency domain. *Comput Electr Eng.* 2018;71:398–407. doi:10.1016/j.compeleceng.2018.07.051

30. Rebouças Filho PP, Sarmento RM, Holanda GB, de Alencar Lima D. New approach to detect and classify stroke in skull CT images via analysis of brain tissue densities. *Comput Methods Programs Biomed.* 2017;148:27–43. doi:10.1016/j.cmpb.2017.06.011

31. Barber PA, Demchuk AM, Zhang J, Buchan AM. Validity and reliability of a quantitative computed tomography score in predicting outcome of hyperacute stroke before thrombolytic therapy. ASPECTS Study Group. Alberta Stroke Programme Early CT Score. *Lancet Lond Engl.* 2000;355(9216):1670–1674. doi:10.1016/s0140–6736(00)02237-6

32. Albers GW, Wald MJ, Mlynash M, et al. Automated calculation of Alberta stroke program early CT Score. *Stroke*. 2019;50(11):3277–3279. doi:10.1161/STROKEAHA.119.026430

33. Seker F, Pfaff J, Nagel S, et al. CT reconstruction levels affect automated and reader-based ASPECTS ratings in acute ischemic stroke. *J Neuroimaging Off J Am Soc Neuroimaging*. 2019;29(1):62–64. doi:10.1111/jon.12562

34. Olive-Gadea M, Martins N, Boned S, et al. Baseline ASPECTS and e-ASPECTS correlation with infarct volume and functional outcome in patients undergoing mechanical thrombectomy. *J Neuroimaging Off J Am Soc Neuroimaging*. 2019;29(2):198–202. doi:10.1111/jon.12564

35. Nagel S, Sinha D, Day D, et al. e-ASPECTS software is non-inferior to neuroradiologists in applying the ASPECT score to computed tomography scans of acute ischemic stroke patients. *Int J Stroke Off J Int Stroke Soc*. 2017;12(6):615–622. doi:10.1177/1747493016681020

36. Guberina N, Dietrich U, Radbruch A, et al. Detection of early infarction signs with machine learning-based diagnosis by means of the Alberta Stroke Program Early CT score (ASPECTS) in the clinical routine. *Neuroradiology*. 2018;60(9):889–901. doi:10.1007/s00234-018-2066-5

37. Herweh C, Ringleb PA, Rauch G, et al. Performance of e-ASPECTS software in comparison to that of stroke physicians on assessing CT scans of acute ischemic stroke patients. *Int J Stroke Off J Int Stroke Soc*. 2016;11(4):438–445. doi:10.1177/1747493016632244

38. Inc iSchemaView. Aneurysm, pulmonary embolism and stroke software platform powered by AI. Accessed August 29, 2022. https://www.rapidai.com

39. Lansberg MG, Straka M, Kemp S, et al. MRI profile and response to endovascular reperfusion after stroke (DEFUSE 2): a prospective cohort study. *Lancet Neurol*. 2012;11(10):860–867. doi:10.1016/S1474-4422(12)70203-X

40. Albers GW, Marks MP, Kemp S, et al. Thrombectomy for stroke at 6 to 16 hours with selection by perfusion imaging. *N Engl J Med*. 2018;378(8):708–718. doi:10.1056/NEJMoa1713973

41. Austein F, Riedel C, Kerby T, et al. Comparison of perfusion CT software to predict the final infarct volume after thrombectomy. *Stroke*. 2016;47(9):2311–2317. doi:10.1161/STROKEAHA.116.013147

42. Campbell BCV, Mitchell PJ, Kleinig TJ, et al. Endovascular therapy for ischemic stroke with perfusion-imaging selection. *N Engl J Med*. 2015;372(11):1009–1018. doi:10.1056/NEJMoa1414792

43. Saver JL, Goyal M, Bonafe A, et al. Stent-retriever thrombectomy after intravenous t-PA vs. t-PA alone in stroke. *N Engl J Med*. 2015;372(24):2285–2295. doi:10.1056/NEJMoa1415061

44. Lansberg MG, Christensen S, Kemp S, et al. Computed tomographic perfusion to predict response to recanalization in ischemic stroke. *Ann Neurol*. 2017;81(6):849–856. doi:10.1002/ana.24953

45. Nogueira RG, Jadhav AP, Haussen DC, et al. Thrombectomy 6 to 24 hours after stroke with a mismatch between deficit and infarct. *N Engl J Med*. 2018;378(1):11–21. doi:10.1056/NEJMoa1706442

46. Chatterjee A, Somayaji NR, Kabakis IM. Abstract WMP16: Artificial intelligence detection of cerebrovascular large vessel occlusion - nine month, 650 patient evaluation of the diagnostic accuracy and performance of the Viz.ai LVO algorithm. *Stroke*. 50(Suppl_1):AWMP16-AWMP16. doi:10.1161/str.50.suppl_1.WMP16

47. G R, Cm B, M B, et al. Automated large artery occlusion detection in stroke: A single-center validation study of an artificial intelligence algorithm. *Cerebrovasc Dis Basel Switz*. 2022;51(2). doi:10.1159/000519125

48. Grunwald IQ, Kulikovski J, Reith W, et al. Collateral automation for triage in stroke: Evaluating automated scoring of collaterals in acute stroke on computed tomography scans. *Cerebrovasc Dis Basel Switz*. 2019;47(5–6):217–222. doi:10.1159/000500076

49. Purrucker JC, Mattern N, Herweh C, et al. Electronic Alberta stroke program early CT score change and functional outcome in a drip-and-ship stroke service. *J Neurointerventional Surg.* 2020;12(3):252–255. doi:10.1136/neurintsurg-2019–015134

50. Seker F, Pfaff JAR, Mokli Y, et al. Diagnostic accuracy of automated occlusion detection in CT angiography using e-CTA. *Int J Stroke Off J Int Stroke Soc.* 2022;17(1):77–82. doi:10.1177/1747493021992592

51. Verdolotti T, Pilato F, Cottonaro S, et al. ColorViz, a new and rapid tool for assessing collateral circulation during stroke. *Brain Sci.* 2020;10(11):882. doi:10.3390/brainsci10110882

52. Maier O, Menze BH, von der Gablentz J, et al. ISLES 2015- A public evaluation benchmark for ischemic stroke lesion segmentation from multispectral MRI. *Med Image Anal.* 2017;35:250–269. doi:10.1016/j.media.2016.07.009

53. Karthik R, Gupta U, Jha A, Rajalakshmi R, Menaka R. A deep supervised approach for ischemic lesion segmentation from multimodal MRI using Fully Convolutional Network. *Appl Soft Comput.* 2019;84:105685. doi:10.1016/j.asoc.2019.105685

54. Jørgensen HS, Nakayama H, Raaschou HO, Olsen TS. Intracerebral hemorrhage versus infarction: Stroke severity, risk factors, and prognosis. *Ann Neurol.* 1995;38(1):45–50. doi:10.1002/ana.410380110

55. Bentley P, Ganesalingam J, Carlton Jones AL, et al. Prediction of stroke thrombolysis outcome using CT brain machine learning. *NeuroImage Clin.* 2014;4:635–640. doi:10.1016/j.nicl.2014.02.003

56. Liu J, Xu H, Chen Q, et al. Prediction of hematoma expansion in spontaneous intracerebral hemorrhage using support vector machine. *EBioMedicine.* 2019;43:454–459. doi:10.1016/j.ebiom.2019.04.040

57. Hilbert A, Ramos LA, van Os HJA, et al. Data-efficient deep learning of radiological image data for outcome prediction after endovascular treatment of patients with acute ischemic stroke. *Comput Biol Med.* 2019;115:103516. doi:10.1016/j.compbiomed.2019.103516

58. Hope TMH, Seghier ML, Leff AP, Price CJ. Predicting outcome and recovery after stroke with lesions extracted from MRI images. *NeuroImage Clin.* 2013;2:424–433. doi:10.1016/j.nicl.2013.03.005

59. Rondina JM, Filippone M, Girolami M, Ward NS. Decoding post-stroke motor function from structural brain imaging. *NeuroImage Clin.* 2016;12:372–380. doi:10.1016/j.nicl.2016.07.014

60. Rehani B, Ammanuel SG, Zhang Y, et al. A new era of extended time window acute stroke interventions guided by imaging. *The Neurohospitalist.* 2020;10(1):29–37. doi:10.1177/1941874419870701

61. Leira EC, Muir KW. Extend trial. *Stroke.* 2019;50(9):2637–2639. doi:10.1161/STROKEAHA.119.026249

62. Miller JB, Heitsch L, Madsen TE, et al. The extended treatment window's impact on emergency systems of care for acute stroke. *Acad Emerg Med Off J Soc Acad Emerg Med.* 2019;26(7):744–751. doi:10.1111/acem.13698

63. Al-Kawaz M, Primiani C, Urrutia V, Hui F. Impact of RapidAI mobile application on treatment times in patients with large vessel occlusion. *J NeuroInterventional Surg.* 2022;14(3):233–236. doi:10.1136/neurintsurg-2021–017365

64. van Leeuwen KG, Meijer FJA, Schalekamp S, et al. Cost-effectiveness of artificial intelligence aided vessel occlusion detection in acute stroke: An early health technology assessment. *Insights Imaging.* 2021;12(1):133. doi:10.1186/s13244-021-01077-4

65. Gao L, Bivard A, Parsons M, et al. Real-world cost-effectiveness of late time window thrombectomy for patients with ischemic stroke. *Front Neurol.* 2021;12:780894. doi:10.3389/fneur.2021.780894

66. Boltyenkov AT, Martinez G, Pandya A, et al. Cost-consequence analysis of advanced imaging in acute ischemic stroke care. *Front Neurol*. 2021;12. Accessed August 29, 2022. https://www.frontiersin.org/articles/10.3389/fneur.2021.774657

67. Yamashita R, Nishio M, Do RKG, Togashi K. Convolutional neural networks: An overview and application in radiology. *Insights Imaging*. 2018;9(4):611–629. doi:10.1007/s13244-018-0639-9

68. Zeleňák K, Krajina A, Meyer L, et al. How to improve the management of acute ischemic stroke by modern technologies, artificial intelligence, and new treatment methods. *Life*. 2021;11(6):488. doi:10.3390/life11060488

69. Mokli Y, Pfaff J, Santos DP dos, Herweh C, Nagel S. Computer-aided imaging analysis in acute ischemic stroke – background and clinical applications. *Neurol Res Pract*. 2019;1. doi:10.1186/s42466-019-0028-y

Applications of Machine Learning and Deep Learning Models in Brain Imaging Analysis

Alwin Joseph, Chandra J, Bonny Banerjee,
Madhavi Rangaswamy, and Jayasankara Reddy K

3.1 INTRODUCTION

Brain imaging or neuroimaging is a technique that helps to monitor the brain and study the structure and function of the human nervous system, especially the activities and design of the human brain and their interactions with the help of images and other forms of data. The technological advancements enable improvement in precision diagnostics for various neurological disorders. Neuroimaging is a technique to identify the brain's structure; this helps the doctors understand brain functioning and effectively identify and conclude the type of neurological disorder the patient possesses. Commonly studied neurological disorders including mild cognitive impairment (MCI), autism spectrum disorder (ASD), schizophrenia, Alzheimer's, and epilepsy are reviewed with the use of images obtained from neuroimaging techniques like functional magnetic resonance imaging (fMRI), electroencephalography (EEG), magnetoencephalography (MEG), positron emission tomography (PET), computed tomography (CT) scans, and diffusion tensor imaging (DTI). Most imaging techniques mentioned above are commonly used and employed in analysing the nature of neurological disorders. The modern-day techniques and support systems for processing neuroimages help doctors reach a conclusion regarding the diseases and take it as a second reference option in various situations. The use of neuroimaging as a source of diagnosis has a few challenges. One of the main challenges is understanding and reaching conclusions from the neuroimages.

The modern technologies (machine learning (ML)- and deep-learning (DL)-based algorithms and tools that are evolving) are designed to process the images and gather insights that the doctors presently use as a medium of validation of their findings from the neuroimages. Doctors can use these modern tools to get a second opinion on their results, which can reduce/eliminate the errors in their insights. Multiple studies focus on developing tools and algorithms for processing neuroimages. Analysing the neuroimages is always challenging; diseases often share a typical structure of neurological impacts and very subtle effects, which can easily go unnoticed. Medical practitioners currently take the help of existing computer-aided applications to validate their findings. However, these applications do not accommodate the multiple neuroimages by limiting their functionality to a specific input type.

ML and DL algorithms are used for processing neuroimages, preprocessing the images by extracting the region of interest from the input images, and then processing them to identify various patterns, comparing the states (before and after) for detecting the changes or impact of the disease. ML algorithms, which include support vector machine (SVM), convolutional neural network (CNN), recurrent neural network (RNN), and random forest, are the most commonly used algorithms for developing models and applications for neuroimages. Researchers focus on creating ML models for neuroimage processing and improving the performance of various models created for processing. Researchers also focus on fine-tuning and extracting the features from the neuroimages, making the algorithms work better with the neuroimages for disease identification. Such research focuses on gathering additional information and image processing to make their predictions more accurate and intelligent. This is achieved with the help of a multimodal approach by combining different types of input towards an ML model.

This chapter identifies and summarises some of the recent advancements in research concerning neuroimaging and the applications of ML models for predicting and classifying various neurological disorders with the help of neuroimaging. The chapter will evaluate the different modalities for brain imaging, studying the superior technologies commonly used for imaging. Then we analyse the performance of various ML models developed concerning these modalities. Finally, we discuss the acceptance of these models in the clinical environment.

3.2 BRAIN IMAGING MODALITIES

This section discusses some fundamental neuroimaging techniques that medical practitioners commonly use to diagnose neurological disorders. Along with the image inputs obtained from these techniques, the doctors collect other related data and finally conclude the nature of the neurological disorder. Brain imaging techniques, experimental designs, and data analysis are used to study the functions of brain regions and examine their interactions with other parts of the brain and body [1]. Commonly used brain imaging (neuroimaging) modalities include the following.

1. fMRI

2. EEG

3. MEG

4. PET

5. CT

6. DTI

A detailed description of the need for each imaging modality is described in the subsections below. The central concept behind each modality, the process in which the image is captured, biological factors considered to capture images, and main diseases that can be identified from the imaging modalities are described briefly to understand the various imaging modalities.

3.2.1 Functional Magnetic Resonance Imaging

fMRI is a brain imaging technique focused on generating the brain image based on the brain's blood level and blood flow. fMRI is based on the concept that blood flow and neuron activities are interdependent. The fMRI image depicts changes in deoxyhaemoglobin concentration. This method is employed in cognition studies for clinical applications such as surgical planning, monitoring treatment outcomes, and as a biomarker in pharmacologic and training programmes. Studies now focus on using pattern classification and other statistical methods to obtain complex inferences about cognitive brain states from fMRI data [2]. The fMRI is based on MRI scanning technology and concentrates on the concentration and properties of oxygen-rich blood, designed to capture the functional changes in the brain due to neuro activities. fMRI can identify epilepsy, stroke, Alzheimer's disease, and multiple sclerosis [3]. Many prominent neurological disorders are identified and traced with the help of fMRI images and other brain imaging techniques.

fMRI helps to determine which part of the brain is active and functioning, mainly concerning a given task. The active part of the brain is tracked with the help of blood movement in the brain. The movement of atoms and molecules can be followed because they have some magnetic resonance, and while they move they emit tiny radio waves that contain protons. The brain activity is observed with the help of the oxygen in haemoglobin; where the activity of the brain is happening, the oxygen from haemoglobin gets used up, and hence we can track the movement of blood. The fMRI scan is a painless and harmless technique that regularly monitors patients under treatment. More about fMRI imaging can be found in [4–6].

3.2.2 Electroencephalography

EEG is another type of brain imaging technique focused on capturing the electrical activity in the brain. EEG is beneficial for evaluating patients with suspected seizures, epilepsy, and unusual spells [5]. EEG is used to assess the integrity of early sensory processing in normal individuals and clinical populations, such as individuals with schizophrenia [6]. The brain activities monitored based on the electrical activity are done with the help of electrodes/metal discs. Brain cell communication is captured through wavy lines or EEG recordings [7]. EEG is effective in capturing the brain's activity due to some spontaneous changes over some time. Epilepsy is a major neurological disorder that can be detected with the help of EEG signals. Other disorders like sleep disorders, anestesia, etc., and the diagnosis of stroke and tumour also use the EEG readings.

EEG helps in tracking the abnormalities in the brain with the help of monitoring the electrical activity in the brain. Electrodes with small metal discs and tin wires are pasted into the scalp to detect the electrical charges from the brain cell activity. The tracked charges are amplified and printed on a paper/computer screen and then used for analysis. EEG explicitly measures the electrical activity to stimulate certain conditions during the test. It helps easily track neurological disorders, including epilepsy, Alzheimer's, narcolepsy, and stroke. EEG is also a safe procedure for brain imaging. More about EEG imaging can be found in [8–11].

3.2.3 Magnetoencephalography

MEG is another type of brain imaging technique that measures the magnetic field generated by the electrical activity of the neurons and electrical currents in the brain [12, 13]. The magnetic fields and interferences produced by the human brain are captured with the help of MEG imaging by using sensitive magnetometers. MEG results are used along with fMRI images for more precise and accurate measurements in the case of identifying brain functions and blood flow. MEG data can also be used for classifying disorders like multiple sclerosis, Alzheimer's, and schizophrenia. Researchers can distinguish the MEG imaging of patients and healthy people as part of the research [14]. MEG is hence a vital technique to finalise various neurological disorders.

MEG imaging helps investigate the brain's activity to precision in milliseconds. MEG works with the concept of electrochemical properties of the neurons that facilitate the flow of charged ions through the cells and capture and measure the electromagnetic fields in the brain. MEG can measure the neurons' electromagnetic fields with the help of superconducting sensors. MEG can show the absolute neuronal activity in the brain. The data captured by MEG and fMRI complement each other as both are associated with measuring the activity in the brain. The MEG data is used to arrive at the exact conclusion related to various disorders. More about MEG imaging and processing can be found in [15–19, 13].

3.2.4 Positron Emission Tomography

PET is an imaging technique that helps track the metabolic/biochemical functions of the tissues and organs with the help of radioactive radiotracers. PET uses the help of a radioactive drug to capture the normal and abnormal metabolic activity [20]. PET effectively captures the metabolic changes related to any body region and helps diagnose diseases effectively using other imaging techniques. PET scans effectively detect different types of cancer, heart diseases, and brain disorders. The major brain disorders that can be tracked with the help of PET include Alzheimer's, seizures, Parkinson's disease (PD), epilepsy, strokes, and tumours.

PET imaging helps obtain a 3D image of the functional properties of the brain. It is based on the nuclear medicine technique, which requires the patient to get injected with a radioactive material (sugar tracer/fluorodeoxyglucose) into the bloodstream. The ring of detectors outside the head can detect the gamma-rays emitted by the tracer injected into the parts of the brain/body under observation. The regions of the brain that get the maximum volume of blood have the most gamma-rays, and the scanner detects these areas, and then they are computed and displayed. PET imaging is mainly used for monitoring visual problems, tumours, and metabolic processes. Single-Photon Emission Computerized Tomography (SPECT) is a variation in PET which is faster than PET. The patients who undergo PET imaging need to fast before the scan, while in SPECT, the patient need not fast. More details of PET scans can be obtained from [4, 20–23].

3.2.5 CT Scan

Computerised tomography (CT) scan is an imaging technique that focuses on obtaining detailed images of any part of the human body. CT scans are performed on special machines with the help of X-rays, by creating slices of the body part to be scanned and then combining it into a 3D structure to identify basic structures, possible tumours, and other abnormalities [24]. A CT scan is done on the brain or head to collect the details for detecting disorders like stroke, tumours, haemorrhages, and bone trauma. Removal of artefacts is an essential process while processing CT scan images. CNNs use different types of encoders like the auto-encoder, which is based on a prominent ML algorithm that is used to learn about CT images [25]; SVM and random forest algorithms perform better for the classification of stroke from CT images [26, 27]. A CT scan is a well-known imaging technique for diagnosing various diseases, accidents, and neurological disorders.

A CT scan uses the help of X-rays to image the brain's structure with details, including blood perfusion. A CT scan can provide 2D and 3D images of the scanned region. The CT image can reveal underdeveloped parts of the brain, sites of injury, tumours, and infections. The CT scan can show detailed images of any body part, including bones, muscles, fat, organs, and blood vessels. Since a CT scan uses X-rays that emit radiation, the patient who undergoes a CT scan has a risk of developing cancer. There are diet restrictions before taking a CT scan. More details of CT scan and ML algorithms that are available for processing CT scan images can be found in [26, 28–31].

3.2.6 Diffusion Tensor Imaging

DTI is an imaging technique based on the concepts of MRI that is used for identifying and tracking microstructural changes, including the diffusion of water in the tissues. This technique is commonly used for characterising the magnitude, degree of anisotropy, and orientation of directional diffusion [32]. DTI imaging is used to capture the white matter substance of the brain in a process called tractography. The resultant image obtained from the scan is converted into RGB colour with a brightness value and viewed with the help of glyphs, which is a small 3D representation of the scanned tensor [33]. The analysis and detection of tensors are done with the help of mathematical concepts, including linear algebra, matrix, and vector mathematics. Neurological disorders like multiple sclerosis,PD, Alzheimer's, epilepsy, and strokes can be detected with the help of the DTI imaging technique.

DTI is a form of MRI to observe the brain's functions and can be observed as they occur. The DTI measures the diffusion of water through the brain tissues. DTI is commonly used to image the white matter in the brain. The DTI can image the neural impulses and how they travel in the brain. DTI is used primarily for the identification of tumours, abnormalities in the brain concerning epilepsy, and other disorders. DTI imaging is also harmless and it takes time to generate the images. ML algorithms are applied to DTI images to process and analyse the imaging result. More details of DTI can be found in [34–37].

These are prominent and widely used imaging techniques for capturing the data for the prognosis of various neurological disorders. The use of technology is limited to analysing these data due to the complex nature of the images and the difference in how the data is captured and processed. The images and the data captured through the image techniques require preprocessing and removing noise from these images. Removal of artefacts and segmentation for extracting the area of interest are some common procedures done on the data of these imaging techniques. Each imaging technique aims to provide detailed information about the part of the body for the analysis and detection of diseases. However, most imaging techniques mentioned in the chapter are closely associated and used in studying the brain and neurological disorders.

Table 3.1 summarises and compares the various neuroimaging techniques used for capturing the neurological data for the prognosis of neurological disorders. A detailed comparison of the techniques with some fundamental differences is mentioned in the table, giving a clear idea of the techniques and their features. The main categories of comparison include measurement, the cost involved in the technique, accuracy of the data, safety of the technique, and the type of signal the imaging technique can capture. Each technique is different from the other and has specific functions to perform in diagnosing various neurological disorders, considering the results of these brain imaging techniques before confirming a brain/neurological disorder.

Table 3.2 summarises the commonly worked neurological disorders with the nature of input brain image modalities. Diseases like epilepsy, stroke, Alzheimer's disease, multiple sclerosis, schizophrenia, Parkinson's, and tumours are studied with the help of different

TABLE 3.1 Comparison of brain imaging techniques

Types of data	fMRI	EEG	MEG	PET	CT	DTI
Measurement	Haemodynamic activity	Brain activity	The magnetic activity of the brain	Perfusion, metabolism, and neurotransmitter dynamics	Brain structure	Fibre tracks
Cost involved	High	Low	High	High	Low	High
Accuracy of the data	High	Low	Medium	High	Low	High
Safety	High	High	Low	Low	Low	High
Signal type	Metabolic	Electrical	Magnetic	Electrical	X-rays	Metabolic

TABLE 3.2   Neuroimage modalities and disorders

Brain image modality	Neurological disorders
fMRI	Epilepsy, stroke, Alzheimer's disease, multiple sclerosis, schizophrenia
EEG	Epilepsy, Alzheimer's, narcolepsy, stroke, seizure disorders, tumours, dementia
MEG	Parkinson's disease, Alzheimer's disease, schizophrenia, multiple sclerosis
PET	Alzheimer's disease, seizures, Parkinson's disease, epilepsy, stroke, tumours, Huntington's disease, multiple sclerosis, and dementias
CT	Stroke, tumour, haemorrhages, epilepsy
DTI	Multiple sclerosis, Parkinson's disease, Alzheimer's disease, epilepsy, stroke, dementia

brain imaging techniques. The doctors confirm the various disorders if the disorder is detected by more than one imaging modality. This is because the nature of changes and the symptoms of different disorders overlap, and detailed observation is required to conclude the actual disease. This is one of the main risks that doctors face in the adoption of technologies with artificial intelligence (AI) and ML; in some cases, AI tools can assist doctors in confirming the diseases based on a detailed study of the imaging data. The doctors take confirmation from multiple imaging techniques to verify the existence of a neurological disorder. Besides the data from the imaging techniques, the doctors need to analyse various other parameters to conclude the neurological disorder since most have similar symptoms and impact on the brain. The main challenge of the different imaging techniques is that most of them cannot identify the existence of a neurological disorder alone. The doctors study the combination of test and scan results to conclude the type of neurological disorder a patient possesses. The cost associated with the imaging techniques is another challenging factor limiting the use and application of these techniques in disease detection. The data's accuracy and the method's safety are some of the patients' worries when prescribed these scans or imaging. The patient's life is in danger if the doctor's conclusion is different; hence validation of their findings is an essential factor in the analysis and prognosis of diseases. ML-based tools can be employed to validate the results.

3.3   ML MODELS FOR PROCESSING AND ANALYSING NEUROIMAGING DATA

Researchers are working on various ML algorithms to process and analyse neuroimaging data for the prognosis of neurological disorders. ML can effectively identify patterns from multiple data sources and help diagnose, treat, and predict complications, especially in patients with neurological disorders. The main approaches the research performs are preparing the data with the help of preprocessing steps and cleaning the data; once the data is adequately made, they then apply ML techniques to learn from these data, and by studying the features of the algorithms are trained to perform classification of the input data to map with a neurological disorder or predict any of the related neurological disorder exists in the patient.

This section covers the AI-ML models that various researchers have applied/developed for the classification/prediction of various neurological disorders from the different neuroimaging modalities. The study could identify various commonly used ML algorithms for the prognosis of various neurological diseases. The ML algorithms used for various brain imaging modalities are listed and described in the following sections.

3.3.1 ML Models for fMRI

ML models are applied to fMRI images that are used to capture brain activity and functional connectivity; the ML models are applied to study various features of these imaging data. This includes the study of the brain concerning hunger/satiety [33], where the study was based on SVM along with various feature selection techniques. An SVM (SNP-SVM, Voxel-SVM, ICA-SVM) model is created to classify people with schizophrenia as healthy people [38]. Supervised ML algorithms, including regression models (ridge regression, LASSO regression, elastic-net regression, logistic regression), SVM (linear SVM, kernelized SVM), decision trees (random forest, gradient-tree boosting), DL techniques (fully connected network, CNNs) are used for the analysis of fMRI images for various neurological disorders including Alzheimer's, MCI, Parkinson's, ALS, schizophrenia, depression, ASD, ADHD, PTSD, and OCD [39]. ASD is diagnosed with fMRI data along with the ML algorithms, including SVM and Artificial Neural Network (ANN), in which SVM performs better [40]. Thus, we can conclude that fMRI is a preferred and commonly used imaging technique for diagnosing various brain-related disorders.

3.3.2 ML Models for EEG

EEG is a brain imaging technique where the brain's signals are captured and analysed for various use cases. EEG data is used with multiple ML algorithms, including deep neural network (DNN), CNN, LSTM, and CNN-LSTM; with the a dataset for emotion analysis using eeg, physiological and video signals (DEAP) dataset, the work was for emotion recognition from EEG signals [41]. While applying ML and DL algorithms to EEG data, wavelet transform is the commonly used technique for feature extraction [42]. While working with EEG signals, the main challenge involved is removing the unwanted noise signals, which significantly impact EEG models' performance. A CNN-based model that preprocessed the EEG signals using RNN and Gated Recurrent Unit (GRU) techniques could achieve 100% accuracy for CNN to classify epilepsy disorders using Bonn and MIT datasets [43]. Neurological diseases such as Alzheimer's (LDA, QDA, MLP, SVM, RF), epilepsy (LS-SVM, SVM, RBF, KNN, naive Bayes, MLP, backpropagation, PCA+ random forest, CNN), and ADHD (SVM, LDA, MLP, SVM, KNN, RF, AdaBoost, NB, LR, CNN) can be detected using EEG signals [44]. The common artefacts that arise with EEG signals include physiological (EOG, EMG, ECG) and non-physiological (instrumental, interference, movements).

3.3.3 ML Models for MEG

MEG is a kind of functional neuroimaging technique which can be used to understand brain functions. PD and Alzheimer's are commonly studied with MEG imaging techniques, which can quickly identify the brain's abnormal activity and disturbed connectivity [19]. MEG data is passed to DNN to diagnose neurological disorders (trained MNet) [45]. Neurological disorders can be classified using pattern recognition and DL techniques. Along with PD and AD, epilepsy can also be detected, and MEG signals with ML can improve treatments for epilepsy [46]. CNN can be used to infer brain states from MEG measurements [47]. Apart from detecting neurological disorders, MEG imaging is applied to study a wide range of other diseases, where the MEG data is used as a test for confirming various conditions.

3.3.4 ML Models for PET

PET is a brain imaging technique closely associated with nuclear medicine that tracks the brain with the help of photons and image reconstruction; PET imaging provides details of the brain concerning perfusion, metabolism, and neurotransmitter dynamics. ML techniques are applied to PET to generate qualitative data [48]. PET data is used to classify neurological disorders like MCI, AD, epilepsy, and tumours [49]. ML algorithms like multi-kernel SVM, random forest, wmSRC, and Gaussian process work to classify Alzheimer's diseases from PET imaging modality [50]. PET images are also used for studying various other disorders.

3.3.5 ML Models for CT Scan

The CT scan is used in identifying and for the prognosis of a wide range of diseases using imaging to study the brain's structure. Strokes are identified with the help of the CT imaging modality; commonly used and identified ML approaches include ANN, SVM, adaptive boosting, and DCNN [51].

3.3.6 ML Models for DTI

DTI modality of neuroimaging helps identify neurological disorders; DTI mainly tracks the fibre tracts in the brain. The commonly studied ML algorithms and DTI data include Gaussian SVM and multi-kernel SVM with Alzheimer's disease classification. Decision tree is used along with DTI imaging for the classification of autism. Parkinson's disorders can be identified with SVM, bootstrap, multinomial logit, and Gaussian SVM ML models [50].

Table 3.3 summarises the commonly used ML algorithms for neuroimaging data analysis and processing. This helps in the analysis and detection of various neurological disorders. The data is processed by removing unwanted data, noise, and artefacts for applying various ML algorithms. From Table 3.3, we can conclude that most imaging modalities are processed and used by the SVM algorithm. Apart from SVM, other ML algorithms are applied by various researchers. However, the results and study of such algorithms are limited.

TABLE 3.3   Neuroimage modalities and commonly used ML algorithms

Brain image modality	AI/ML algorithms
fMRI	SVM, regression, decision trees, ANN, CNN
EEG	LDA, MLP, SVM, RF, RBF, KNN, NB, PCA, RF
MEG	DNN, CNN
PET	SVM, RF
CT	ANN, SVM, CNN, DCNN
DTI	SVM, decision tree, random forest

Removal of artefacts is integral to preprocessing and preparing neuroimaging data before analysis. The preprocessing parts fine-tune the obtained neuroimage and make it the best fit for the study. ICA-AROMA can be used with fMRI data to remove motion artefacts and other structured noise [52]. Removing artefacts and cleaning the data is an integral part of processing the brain imaging data. The preprocessed data help the effective processing of the images by improving the results of the models.

3.4 PIPELINES FOR CLINICAL PERSPECTIVES

It is difficult to adopt ML models and applications created for various neurological disorders in the clinical setting; this is due to the possibility of errors and the various use cases. ML models can only be used as a secondary option by doctors as it is related to multiple factors [53].

With the advancement in technology in science and medicine, various brain imaging techniques have emerged in neuroscience. Techniques such as CT scan, fMRI, EEG, etc., use elaborate scientific methods to record brain structures and functions. The major brain imaging techniques are EEG, which is a tool used to measure the electrical activity in the brain; fMRI, which is a common neuroimaging technique to explore the brain structures; and CT scans which are used to produce detailed images including the bones, muscles, fat, blood vessels, etc. These imaging techniques act as catalysts in research and practice, providing more evidence to theories and pathology. They are also used as biomarkers, where underlying causes and predictions in the pathology are understood, to create effective treatment. Consequently, brain imaging techniques are used to monitor and validate the interventions given, facilitating a significant impact.

Despite their advantages, there remain challenges in interpreting data from multiple sources. These imaging techniques have changed the direction of treatment and research in neuroscience. However, even with their strengths, there are some challenges that researchers and clinicians face when interpreting data connected to brain imaging. First, each imaging technique is curated to measure a specific brain feature, so integrating information would be time-consuming and difficult. Second, the methods have a unique format for acquiring and storing data. The interpretation is based on age and gender, making it more complex and requiring norms. Third, most research needs data to be present in a numerical and quantitative form, which requires elaborate conversions by trained professionals. This would increase the time and human resources needed to interpret the information. Lastly, this modality makes it challenging to compare data in longitudinal studies.

3.5 DISCUSSION

Various challenges and problems are associated with each neurological disorder. The main challenge of neuroimage processing is the images generated from different imaging platforms. Also, patient data, which is personal, is not available for the researchers to work on improving the algorithms they create to accommodate extensive scale usage of the models for classification and predictions. Creating a model that accommodates the various neuroimaging modalities helps reach proper conclusions faster and more effectively. The

ML algorithms and models must be made to accommodate multiple modalities to finalise and detect neurological disorders. The solution to improving the integration of imaging techniques thus lies in the advancement of AI and ML techniques. Incorporating multiple modalities of neuroimages for the model has to be carefully done with high intelligence as disease detection does not require inputs from all the imaging techniques. Also, the external patient factors are to be considered. The development of such complicated models that accommodate this kind of intelligent model and technique will ease the work of doctors in concluding the presence of diseases and provide more revelations in neuroscience.

3.6 CONCLUSIONS

This chapter identifies the standard neuroimaging techniques commonly used to identify diseases by studying the patterns in the brain. The widely used ML algorithms for processing and analysing brain imaging modalities are also discussed in detail. The chapter summarises the work carried out in the area and whether further improvements are required for various models created for the analysis. The study could identify that fMRI, EEG, MEG, PET, CT, and DTI are the main imaging modalities clinicians use to identify various neurological disorders. The commonly studied neurological/brain-related disorders include epilepsy, stroke, Alzheimer's disease, multiple sclerosis, schizophrenia, PD, and tumours. The ML algorithms help analyse and classify the input data from various modalities. Various processing techniques are designed to capture the exact details from the different modalities. The ML algorithms that work better with multiple modalities for classifying and identifying neurological disorders include MLP, SVM, RF, DT, ANN, CNN, and DCNN.

REFERENCES

[1] G. Xue, X. U. E. Gui, C. Chen, L. U. Zhong-Lin, and Q. Dong, "Brain imaging techniques and their applications in decision-making research," *Acta Psychol. Sin.*, vol. 42, no. 1. pp. 120–137, 2010. doi: 10.3724/sp.j.1041.2010.00120.

[2] G. H. Glover, "Overview of functional magnetic resonance imaging," *Neurosurg. Clin. N. Am.*, vol. 22, no. 2, pp. 133–139, vii, Apr. 2011, doi: 10.1016/j.nec.2010.11.001.

[3] T. Auer, A. Schwarcz, R. A. Horváth, P. Barsi, and J. Janszky, "Functional magnetic resonance imaging in neurology," *Ideggyogy. Sz.*, vol. 61, no. 1–2, pp. 16–23, Jan. 2008, [Online]. Available: https://www.ncbi.nlm.nih.gov/pubmed/18372771

[4] Anthea Wright, "Brain scanning techniques (CT, MRI, fMRI, PET, SPECT, DTI, DOT)," https://psicoterapiabilbao.es/wp-content/uploads/2015/12/Brain_scanning_techniques.pdf (accessed Jul. 26, 2022).

[5] "Website." Britton JW, Frey LC, Hopp JL et al., authors; St. Louis EK, Frey LC, editors. *Electroencephalography (EEG): An Introductory Text and Atlas of Normal and Abnormal Findings in Adults, Children, and Infants [Internet].* Chicago, IL: American Epilepsy Society; 2016. https://www.ncbi.nlm.nih.gov/books/NBK390354/

[6] G. A. Light *et al.*, "Electroencephalography (EEG) and Event-Related Potentials (ERPs) with human participants," *Curr. Protoc. Neurosci.*, vol. Chapter 6, p. Unit 6.25.1–24, July 2010, doi: 10.1002/0471142301.ns0625s52.

[7] "EEG (electroencephalogram)," May 11, 2022. https://www.mayoclinic.org/tests-procedures/eeg/about/pac-20393875 (accessed July 19, 2022).

[8] "Electroencephalogram (EEG)," Aug. 08, 2021. https://www.hopkinsmedicine.org/health/treatment-tests-and-therapies/electroencephalogram-eeg (accessed July 26, 2022).

[9] S. Siuly, Y. Li, and Y. Zhang, *EEG Signal Analysis and Classification: Techniques and Applications*. Springer, 2017. [Online]. Available: https://play.google.com/store/books/details?id=NS7VDQAAQBAJ

[10] W. Y. Leong, *EEG Signal Processing: Feature Extraction, Selection and Classification Methods*. Healthcare Technologies, 2019. [Online]. Available: https://books.google.com/books/about/EEG_Signal_Processing.html?hl=&id=IOOUtQEACAAJ

[11] L. Hu and Z. Zhang, *EEG Signal Processing and Feature Extraction*. Springer Nature, 2019. [Online]. Available: https://play.google.com/store/books/details?id=1dW1DwAAQBAJ

[12] S. P. Singh, "Magnetoencephalography: Basic principles," *Ann. Indian Acad. Neurol.*, vol. 17, no. Suppl 1, pp. S107–S112, Mar. 2014, doi: 10.4103/0972-2327.128676.

[13] Radiological Society of North America (RSNA) and American College of Radiology (ACR), "Magnetoencephalography," *Radiologyinfo.org*. https://www.radiologyinfo.org/en/info/meg (accessed July 19, 2022).

[14] A. P. Georgopoulos *et al.*, "Synchronous neural interactions assessed by magnetoencephalography: A functional biomarker for brain disorders," *Journal of Neural Engineering*, vol. 4, no. 4. pp. 349–355, 2007. doi: 10.1088/1741-2560/4/4/001.

[15] "What is Magnetoencephalography (MEG)?," https://ilabs.uw.edu/what-magnetoencephalography-meg/ (accessed July 26, 2022).

[16] A. Aboughazala, *Multidimensional Signal Processing of EEG and MEG Signals*. 2018. [Online]. Available: https://books.google.com/books/about/Multidimensional_Signal_Processing_of_EE.html?hl=&id=GqaNswEACAAJ

[17] R. B. Clarke, *Signal Processing for Magnetoencephalography*. 2010. [Online]. Available: https://books.google.com/books/about/Signal_Processing_for_Magnetoencephalogr.html?hl=&id=DuWukQEACAAJ

[18] R. Vigario, J. Sarela, V. Jousmiki, M. Hamalainen, and E. Oja, "Independent component approach to the analysis of EEG and MEG recordings," *IEEE Transactions on Biomedical Engineering*, vol. 47, no. 5. pp. 589–593, 2000. doi: 10.1109/10.841330.

[19] C. J. Stam, "Use of magnetoencephalography (MEG) to study functional brain networks in neurodegenerative disorders," *J. Neurol. Sci.*, vol. 289, no. 1–2, pp. 128–134, Feb. 2010, doi: 10.1016/j.jns.2009.08.028.

[20] "Positron emission tomography scan," Aug. 10, 2021. https://www.mayoclinic.org/tests-procedures/pet-scan/about/pac-20385078 (accessed Jul. 20, 2022).

[21] "Positron emission tomography," *Handbook of Physics in Medicine and Biology*. pp. 365–370, 2010. doi: 10.1201/9781420075250-36.

[22] J. M. Ollinger and J. A. Fessler, "Positron-emission tomography," *IEEE Signal Processing Magazine*, vol. 14, no. 1. pp. 43–55, 1997. doi: 10.1109/79.560323.

[23] "Website," https://doi.org/10.1002/ana.410220408

[24] "Computed Tomography (CT)," https://www.nibib.nih.gov/science-education/science-topics/computed-tomography-ct (accessed July 20, 2022).

[25] G. Zhu, B. Jiang, L. Tong, Y. Xie, G. Zaharchuk, and M. Wintermark, "Applications of deep learning to neuro-imaging techniques," *Front. Neurol.*, vol. 10, p. 869, Aug. 2019, doi: 10.3389/fneur.2019.00869.

[26] M. S. Sirsat, E. Fermé, and J. Câmara, "Machine learning for brain stroke: A review," *Journal of Stroke and Cerebrovascular Diseases*, vol. 29, no. 10. p. 105162, 2020. doi: 10.1016/j.jstrokecerebrovasdis.2020.105162.

[27] P. Bentley *et al.*, "Prediction of stroke thrombolysis outcome using CT brain machine learning," *Neuroimage Clin*, vol. 4, pp. 635–640, Mar. 2014, doi: 10.1016/j.nicl.2014.02.003.

[28] W. Lanksch, E. Kazner, and T. Grumme, "Basic principles of computed tomography," *Computed Tomography in Head Injuries.* pp. 1–16, 1979. doi: 10.1007/978-3-642-67421-1_1.

[29] L. Itu *et al.*, "A machine-learning approach for computation of fractional flow reserve from coronary computed tomography," *J. Appl. Physiol.*, vol. 121, no. 1, pp. 42–52, July 2016, doi: 10.1152/japplphysiol.00752.2015.

[30] R. L. Draelos *et al.*, "Machine-learning-based multiple abnormality prediction with large-scale chest computed tomography volumes," *Med. Image Anal.*, vol. 67, p. 101857, Jan. 2021, doi: 10.1016/j.media.2020.101857.

[31] A. M. Fischer *et al.*, "Machine learning/Deep neuronal network: Routine application in chest computed tomography and workflow considerations," *J. Thorac. Imaging*, vol. 35 Suppl 1, pp. S21–S27, May 2020, doi: 10.1097/RTI.0000000000000498.

[32] A. L. Alexander, J. E. Lee, M. Lazar, and A. S. Field, "Diffusion tensor imaging of the brain," *Neurotherapeutics*, vol. 4, no. 3, pp. 316–329, Jul. 2007, doi: 10.1016/j.nurt.2007.05.011.

[33] L. J. O'Donnell and C.-F. Westin, "An introduction to diffusion tensor image analysis," *Neurosurg. Clin. N. Am.*, vol. 22, no. 2, p. 185, Apr. 2011, doi: 10.1016/j.nec.2010.12.004.

[34] J. Ma, X. Yang, F. Xu, and H. Li, "Application of Diffusion Tensor Imaging (DTI) in the Diagnosis of HIV-Associated Neurocognitive Disorder (HAND): A meta-analysis and a system review," *Front. Neurol.*, vol. 13, p. 898191, Jul. 2022, doi: 10.3389/fneur.2022.898191.

[35] "Principle of diffusion tensor imaging," *Introduction to Diffusion Tensor Imaging.* pp. 27–32, 2014. doi: 10.1016/b978-0-12-398398-5.00004-7.

[36] Z. S. Zheng, N. Reggente, E. Lutkenhoff, A. M. Owen, and M. M. Monti, "Disentangling disorders of consciousness: Insights from diffusion tensor imaging and machine learning," *Hum. Brain Mapp.*, vol. 38, no. 1, pp. 431–443, Jan. 2017, doi: 10.1002/hbm.23370.

[37] L. Billeci, A. Badolato, L. Bachi, and A. Tonacci, "Machine learning for the classification of Alzheimer's disease and its prodromal stage using brain diffusion tensor imaging data: A systematic review," *Processes*, vol. 8, no. 9. p. 1071, 2020. doi: 10.3390/pr8091071.

[38] H. Yang, J. Liu, J. Sui, G. Pearlson, and V. D. Calhoun, "A hybrid machine learning method for fusing fMRI and genetic data: Combining both improves classification of schizophrenia," *Front. Hum. Neurosci.*, vol. 0, 2010, doi: 10.3389/fnhum.2010.00192.

[39] "Machine learning in resting-state fMRI analysis," *Magn. Reson. Imaging*, vol. 64, pp. 101–121, Dec. 2019, doi: 10.1016/j.mri.2019.05.031.

[40] C. P. Santana, E. A. de Carvalho, I. D. Rodrigues, G. S. Bastos, A. D. de Souza, and L. L. de Brito, "rs-fMRI and machine learning for ASD diagnosis: A systematic review and meta-analysis," *Sci. Rep.*, vol. 12, no. 1, pp. 1–20, Apr. 2022, doi: 10.1038/s41598-022-09821-6.

[41] Y. Zhang *et al.*, "An investigation of deep learning models for EEG-based emotion recognition," *Front. Neurosci.*, vol. 0, 2020, doi: 10.3389/fnins.2020.622759.

[42] M. Saeidi *et al.*, "Neural decoding of EEG signals with machine learning: A systematic review," *Brain Sciences*, vol. 11, no. 11, p. 1525, Nov. 2021, doi: 10.3390/brainsci11111525.

[43] G. Bouallegue, R. Djemal, S. A. Alshebeili, and H. Aldhalaan, "A dynamic filtering DF-RNN deep-learning-based approach for EEG-based neurological disorders diagnosis," *IEEE Access*, vol. 8. pp. 206992–207007, 2020. doi: 10.1109/access.2020.3037995.

[44] V. Joshi and N. Nanavati, "A review of EEG signal analysis for diagnosis of neurological disorders using machine learning," *Journal of Biomedical Photonics & Engineering*, vol. 7, no. 4. p. 040201, 2021. doi: 10.18287/10.18287/jbpe21.07.040201.

[45] J. Aoe *et al.*, "Automatic diagnosis of neurological diseases using MEG signals with a deep neural network," *Sci. Rep.*, vol. 9, no. 1, p. 5057, Mar. 2019, doi: 10.1038/s41598-019-41500-x.

[46] I. A. Nissen *et al.*, "Localization of the epileptogenic zone using interictal MEG and machine learning in a large cohort of drug-resistant epilepsy patients," *Frontiers in Neurology*, vol. 9. 2018. doi: 10.3389/fneur.2018.00647.

[47] I. Zubarev, R. Zetter, H.-L. Halme, and L. Parkkonen, "Adaptive neural network classifier for decoding MEG signals," *Neuroimage*, vol. 197, pp. 425–434, Aug. 2019, doi: 10.1016/j.neuroimage.2019.04.068.

[48] K. Gong, E. Berg, S. R. Cherry, and J. Qi, "Machine learning in PET: From photon detection to quantitative image reconstruction," *Proceedings of the IEEE*, vol. 108, no. 1. pp. 51–68, 2020. doi: 10.1109/jproc.2019.2936809.

[49] K. Sakai and K. Yamada, "Machine learning studies on major brain diseases: 5-year trends of 2014–2018," *Japanese Journal of Radiology*, vol. 37, no. 1. pp. 34–72, 2019. doi: 10.1007/s11604-018-0794-4.

[50] "Structural neuroimaging as clinical predictor: A review of machine learning applications," *NeuroImage: Clinical*, vol. 20, pp. 506–522, Jan. 2018, doi: 10.1016/j.nicl.2018.08.019.

[51] H. Kamal, V. Lopez, and S. A. Sheth, "Machine learning in acute ischemic stroke neuroimaging," *Frontiers in Neurology*, vol. 9. 2018. doi: 10.3389/fneur.2018.00945.

[52] A. Al-Zubaidi, A. Mertins, M. Heldmann, K. Jauch-Chara, and T. F. Münte, "Machine learning based classification of resting-state fMRI features exemplified by metabolic state (Hunger/Satiety)," *Front. Hum. Neurosci.*, vol. 0, 2019, doi: 10.3389/fnhum.2019.00164.

[53] J. Chandra *et al.*, "Applications of artificial intelligence to neurological disorders: Current technologies and open problems," *Augmenting Neurological Disorder Prediction and Rehabilitation Using Artificial Intelligence*. pp. 243–272, 2022. doi: 10.1016/b978-0-323-90037-9.00005–9.

CHAPTER 4

A Survey on Deep Learning for Neuroimaging-Based Brain Disorder Analysis

Sushil S. Kokare and Revathy V. R.

4.1 INTRODUCTION

Stroke is a one of the serious health problems which causes disability and even death in many cases. The number of cases of stroke has gone up a lot in the past few decades, and now more people than ever are at risk of having a stroke sometime in their life. The majority of the burden caused by stroke (86% of deaths and 89% of disability) occurs in lower- and lower-middle-income countries, posing a significant problem for families with finite resources.

High blood pressure increases the chance of having a stroke, along with factors such as tobacco use, unhealthy diet, alcohol consumption, and obesity. Stroke can lead to significant physical and emotional impacts, including physical disability, communication difficulties, and loss of work and social networks. Quick access to treatment can improve outcomes for stroke survivors.

Recognizing stroke signs such as sudden numbness or weakness in the face, arm, or leg (usually on one side of the body), sudden confusion or difficulty speaking or understanding speech, sudden trouble seeing in one or both eyes, sudden dizziness, loss of balance or coordination, and sudden severe headache with no known cause is crucial. Seeking immediate medical attention can improve outcomes and save lives. The "FAST" (Facial drooping, Arm weakness, Speech difficulties, and Time) approach helps individuals quickly identify a stroke and seek immediate treatment at a hospital.

There are various imaging techniques used for stroke, including computed tomography (CT), CT angiography (CTA), CT perfusion, magnetic resonance imaging (MRI), and MR perfusion. Each method has its own pros and cons. Imaging in stroke CT and MRI is the

DOI: 10.1201/9781003264767-4

backbone of stroke analytics for both research and clinical decision support [10]. Brain imaging, particularly MRI, is utilized in research to comprehend the impact of therapy on the brain and predict rehabilitation results. It offers valuable information beyond what bedside exams can provide [12].

CT scan is a commonly used imaging technique in stroke patients to detect any intracranial hematoma or lesion, and to exclude hemorrhagic stroke. Non-contrast CT (NCCT) is the first imaging technique done to identify calcification and the age of infarction. CTA is performed to identify any vessel occlusion or thrombosis, aneurysm, vasculitis, and dissection. Computed tomography perfusion (CTP) is a diagnostic tool used to assess the blood flow in the brain and identify areas of decreased blood flow, which may indicate stroke or other cerebrovascular diseases. It can detect the ischemic penumbra, which is the area of the brain that is at risk of damage due to decreased blood flow, and the core infarction, which is the area of the brain that has already been damaged. CTP uses X-rays to produce detailed images of the brain, and the data is processed to provide information about cerebral blood volume and flow. However, CTP is not without limitations and can be affected by artifacts and other technical challenges, which can impact the accuracy of the results.

Diffusion-weighted imaging (DWI) is a highly sensitive and accurate medical imaging technique used to detect ischemic stroke in its early stages. It works by measuring the restricted Brownian motion of water molecules in infarcted tissue, which appears as a hypersignal on the DWI image. An additional sequence, called the apparent diffusion coefficient (ADC), is used to differentiate true diffusion restriction from brain edema.

The field of artificial intelligence (AI) technology is rapidly advancing and has various applications in acute stroke imaging, encompassing ischemic and hemorrhage subtypes [38]. Neuroimaging is an important tool for the detection, characterization, and prognostication of acute strokes, including ischemic and hemorrhagic subtypes [38]. Machine learning (ML) and deep learning (DL) subsets of AI are being used in the field of brain stroke to improve diagnosis, treatment, and patient outcomes. The commonly used DL algorithms in medical applications include convolutional neural networks (CNNs) [9].These technologies have the potential to revolutionize the way brain strokes are managed, leading to better patient outcomes.

In terms of predictive modeling, ML algorithms can be trained on large datasets of patient data and imaging studies to identify the risk factors and predict the likelihood of a stroke. This information can be leveraged to target prevention efforts more effectively and reduce the number of strokes that occur.

For stroke diagnosis, CNNs can be used to analyze medical images, such as MRI or CT scans, and assist radiologists in detecting signs of stroke. These algorithms have been trained on large datasets of medical images and have been shown to have high accuracy in detecting strokes. This can improve the speed and accuracy of stroke diagnosis, leading to better patient outcomes. Although DL techniques in medical imaging are still in their initial stages, they have been utilized with great enthusiasm, resulting in significant advancements. These techniques are becoming increasingly popular and have the potential to revolutionize medical imaging, leading to more accurate and efficient diagnoses [16]. DL algorithms have revolutionized computer vision research and led to significant advancements in the analysis of radiologic images [16].

Furthermore, AI and its subset can be utilized in the analysis of patient data and imaging studies to figure out the best treatment options for individual patients. This can enhance patient outcomes by facilitating more individual and effective treatment plans. Additionally, AI algorithms can be used to monitor patients after stroke and assess the effectiveness of their treatment over time. This can help healthcare providers make necessary adjustments to treatment plans and elevate patient results.

In conclusion, AI and its subset (ML and DL) have the potential to transform the way brain strokes are diagnosed, treated, and managed. While these technologies are still in their experimental stages of development, they hold potential for enhancing patient outcomes in the future. The chapter is further divided into Section 4.2 (Search Strategies), Section 4.3 (Magnetic Resonance Imaging), Section 4.4 (Computed Tomography), Section 4.5 (Other than CT & MRI Imaging Modalities), Section 4.6 (Limitations & Future Trends), Section 4.7 (Conclusion), and References.

4.2 SEARCH STRATEGIES

We have collected all the papers from the Google Scholar website. The year-wise distribution of papers is shown in Figure 4.1.

4.3 MAGNETIC RESONANCE IMAGING

MRI is a powerful imaging modality that is commonly utilized to detect and assess stroke. MRI- based neuroimaging can provide detailed information about the extent and severity of the stroke, which can help guide treatment decisions and predict outcomes.

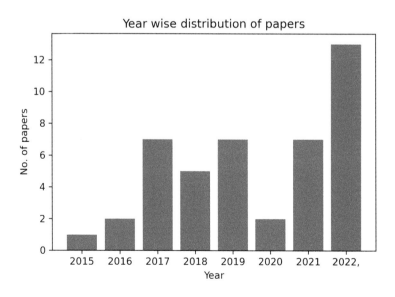

FIGURE 4.1   Year-wise distribution of papers.

MRI offers several benefits over CT for the diagnosis of stroke. MRI is more sensitive than CT in early diagnosis of change in the brain linked to stroke, has better contrast resolution, is safer since it does not use ionizing radiation, and provides multiparametric information about the brain. Additionally, the sensitivity of MRI allows for the detection of stroke up to 24 hours after onset of symptoms, whereas CT can only detect stroke within the first few hours. Overall, MRI is considered the benchmark for stroke diagnosis and evaluation, and is preferred over CT for most stroke patients.

Following are some of the researches that used MRI scans as inputs in order to diagnose stroke.

4.3.1 MRI for Lesion

Automatic lesion identification or segmentation is a critical component of precision medicine when dealing with large datasets of brain imaging. This is because manual lesion segmentation can be time-consuming and prone to inconsistency among different raters, making automated methods indispensable for efficient and reliable analysis [4].

A 3D CNN can capture spatial information from volumetric data, which is crucial for accurate stroke diagnosis, while a 2D CNN cannot; 3D CNN models process a sequence of volumetric images to build a volumetric representation of the data, potentially improving diagnostic accuracy and providing more detailed information about the stroke's extent and location. Lesion segmentation in stroke involves using medical imaging techniques to identify and delineate areas of tissue damage in the brain caused by a stroke. Following this the author in [2] developed an ensemble of 3D multiscale residual U-net and a fully connected network for lesion outcome prediction. The residual U-net model produced successful segmentation outcomes but was subject to artifacts, which are errors or inconsistencies in the segmentation results. While the FCN (fully convolutional network) model incorporated clinical information but produced noisy voxel-wise predictions.

Ensembling the two models improved prediction accuracy and robustness. The ensemble approach performed well in both problems, ranking among the leading submissions in the ISLES (Ischemic Stroke Lesion Segmentation) 2016 Challenge. Lesion segmentation in stroke involves using medical imaging techniques to identify and delineate areas of tissue damage in the brain caused by a stroke. [3] describes a 3D CNN for brain lesion segmentation that includes a dual pathway approach, with the second pathway having higher-level features and the first pathway capturing detailed local appearance. A 3D fully connected conditional random field is used for refinement of the network's soft segmentation. An adaptive solution to class imbalance in segmentation issues is provided by the DeepMedic CNN architecture, and the advantages of using small convolutional kernels in 3D CNNs are also examined. Clinical evaluation of the proposed method on head trauma, brain tumors, and ischemic stroke shows promising results with cutting-edge benchmark performance.

While a simple MRI offers in-depth visualizations of the internal anatomy of the body, a DWI MRI offers an extra perspective on the transfer of water molecules within tissues, which can help to identify certain medical conditions. The authors of paper [8] propose novel DL architecture for automatically recognizing acute ischemic lesions in DWI.

It includes two networks, EDD Net and MUSCLE Net, for detection and false-positive removal. The EDD Net outperforms the baseline CNNs.

MR perfusion is a type of MRI that provides functional information about the blood flow in tissues and organs. This technique can help to identify areas of abnormal blood flow, such as those caused by tumors or strokes [19]. The authors used DeepMedic CNN to segment stroke lesions in MR perfusion imaging. They improved results by 17% using data augmentation with binary closing. Adaptive sampling method for DeepMedic was also proposed. They also concluded that more work is needed for reliable automatic segmentation in clinical environments due to lesion heterogeneity.

The core of an ischemic stroke is the central region of the brain that is immediately affected by the lack of blood flow. This area is typically characterized by severe damage and irreversible cell death, as brain cells require a constant supply of oxygen and glucose to survive whereas the penumbra of an ischemic stroke is the surrounding area of the brain that is still receiving some blood flow, but not enough to function normally. This area is considered to be at risk of progressing to irreversible damage if blood flow is not restored quickly. The authors [21] propose a fully automated method for estimating the core and penumbra in ischemic stroke lesions using MRI, which employs CNNs for semantic segmentation. The experimental validation of the method was conducted using the ISLES 2015 dataset and exhibits generalization capability despite being trained with few annotated samples. The authors conclude that the proposed method provides a unified framework that leverages both diffusion and perfusion maps to perform DL-based segmentation of both core and penumbra regions, yielding accuracy comparable to existing methods.

The [25] paper presents a study on the detection of ischemic stroke lesions using DL object detection networks on brain MRI images. Three networks were tested; faster R-CNN, YOLOv3 (You Only Look Once v3), and SSD (single-shot multibox detector) and SSD had the best precision of 89.77%. The authors provide details on the network architectures and training procedures used. The research can aid in the intelligent-assisted diagnosis and treatment of stroke. Also, [13] article discusses the use of MRI techniques to predict lesion outcome after ischemic stroke. DL models, particularly CNNs, are more accurate than RF ML (random forest ML) in this task. The ISLES team has created a public MRI database for ischemic stroke lesion MRI; this database serves as a benchmark framework that researchers can use to assess the effectiveness of their algorithms against established methods.

ISLES is an international initiative that provides a standardized platform for evaluating algorithms used for classifying ischemic stroke lesions in MRI scans. They have developed a public MRI database and organize challenges to boost accuracy of lesion delineation. The goal is to improve clinical decision-making and patient outcomes. The use of this database and open evaluation system has the capability to elevate the accuracy of lesion outcome prediction and serve as a standard for future research in this field.

Perfusion maps are a type of medical imaging technique that is used to assess the blood flow to different regions of the brain. Perfusion maps are generated by analyzing dynamic contrast-enhanced MRI (DCE-MRI) data, which involves introducing a contrast agent into the bloodstream and then tracking how it flows through the brain over time. Perfusion maps can also be used to guide treatment decisions, such as determining whether a patient is a candidate for thrombolytic therapy (clot-busting drugs) in the case of stroke, or for radiation therapy planning in the case of brain tumors. The next paper [18] explored the use of CNNs for generating perfusion maps in individuals diagnosed with acute ischemic stroke (AIS). The CNN method was rapid and did not necessitate an explicit definition of an arterial input function. The CNN method and the reference method demonstrated strong agreement, and the perfusion maps generated by CNN could be utilized with comparable clinical efficacy. Lesion volumes differed slightly between the two methods, but the CNN method had complete agreement on eligibility for reperfusion treatment. The [15] study examined the use of CNNs for predicting language disorder severity from 3D lesion images in stroke patients. CNNs outperformed conventional ML methods and their performance scaled with the amount of training data. Training data size and image redundancy were crucial elements for accuracy. A hybrid method that combined CNN features with PCA (principal component analysis) image features produced the best results. Overall, DL shows promise for predicting behavioral outcomes from brain imaging data.

4.3.2 MRI for Tissue Fate

Tissue fate refers to the outcome of the brain tissue affected by the interruption of blood flow. The fate of the tissue depends on the duration and severity of the blood flow interruption, as well as the ability of collateral blood vessels to provide alternative sources of blood supply. During a stroke, brain cells begin to die within minutes due to lack of oxygen and nutrients.

[1] Study developed a predictive model of tissue fate in ischemic stroke using a CNN. A CNN was trained using local patches selected at random from the hypoperfusion feature detected in MRI shortly after the onset of symptoms. The CNN was able to accurately forecast tissue fate by taking into account the context of each voxel and modeling the non-linear correlation between Tmax and tissue fate. The study suggests that a relatively simple CNN can be used to accurately predict tissue fate in ischemic stroke at the time of symptom onset. [1] suggests that using a modified 3D CNN, which utilizes the additional information provided by the 3D data of MRI, may increase the predictive power of the model. The [11] article discusses the development and evaluation of different predictive models for final imaging outcome in AIS using MRI data. Three different CNNs were implemented, including CNNTmax, CNNshallow, and CNNdeep. The performance of these models was compared with a generalized linear model. CNNdeep showed superior performance in predicting final outcome compared with other models. Predicted images showed improved contrast and accuracy in distinguishing outcomes based on treatment strategy, thanks to CNNdeep. Compared to a voxel-based model, CNNs offer the advantage of retaining spatial information, which leads to more precise predictions. The performance of the CNN relies on its depth, which can significantly enhance its accuracy. Stroke infarction denotes the demise of cerebral tissue owing to insufficient blood supply triggered by the obstruction of an artery in the brain. The impediment can arise from the development of a blood clot inside an artery located in the brain or from a clot originating elsewhere in the body and reaching the brain. When brain tissue is deprived of oxygen and nutrients, it can quickly become damaged or die, leading to various neurological symptoms such as weakness,

numbness, difficulty speaking, vision problems, and more. The paper [35] explores the use of deep CNNs to predict stroke infarction thickness using primary perfusion data. The proposed model outshines existing systems in terms of accuracy, error rate, and time complexity. The study shows that noninvasive technologies can track stroke illnesses in real time, aiding physicians in determining the severity of treatment. While further research is needed to enhance predictive performance, CNNs offer potential for improving with each patient encounter.

Preventing overfitting is important in DL because it aids in ensuring that the model can generalize effectively to novel and unseen data. Overfitting transpires when a model's complexity surpasses the need to discern meaningful patterns and features from the training data, leading to the model memorizing the data instead of learning to generalize and make accurate predictions on unseen data. When a model overfits, it performs very well on the training data but poorly on new data, which can lead to inaccurate predictions and reduced performance. [7] discusses different strategies to prevent overfitting in DL architectures, such as data augmentation, dropout, and regularization. Transfer learning is also introduced as a way to improve generalization by fine-tuning a pre-trained network on a specific dataset. However, DL techniques for brain MRI are still challenging due to variations in data and small training datasets. There is a need for more robust and unsupervised learning models, besides data augmentation methods that replicate variations found in brain MRI. Transfer learning can be used to share well-performing models among the research community and improve generalization across datasets.

Quad convolutional layers CNN (QCL-CNN) is a DL architecture that uses four convolutional layers to extract features from input images for stroke brain diagnosis. Compared to other CNN models, QCL-CNN may have better feature extraction capabilities, improved discrimination of stroke lesions, reduced overfitting, and faster training and inference times. However, the effectiveness of employing this approach may be contingent on various factors, including the quality of the input data and the availability of suitable computational resources. Overall, QCL-CNN is a promising approach for stroke brain diagnosis that balances model complexity and training efficiency.

The authors of [43] demonstrate the potential of DL techniques in improving the accuracy of brain stroke diagnosis using MRI images by developing a new model QCL-CNN, for classifying different types of brain stroke injuries based on diffusion-weighted magnetic resonance (DW-MR) images, which outperforms other methods like AlexNet, ResNet50, and VGG16. The study used two datasets with two and three classes and achieved high accuracy in classifying hemorrhagic, ischemic, and normal brain images.

4.3.3 Uses of Magnetic Resonance Imaging

Brain imaging is crucial in the diagnosis and understanding of the evolution of AIS. DWI and ADC maps are useful tools for early detection of AIS lesions and differentiating them from stroke mimics. [27, 29] use CNN on ADC. In [27] the authors used only diffusion and ADC information, developing a 3D CNN algorithm to segment stroke lesions and classify subtypes. The proposed method achieved high accuracy for both lesion segmentation and stroke subtype classification. However, the most widely used TOAST (Trial of

Org 10172 in Acute Stroke Treatment) classification system employed in the study has inherent limitations in accurately categorizing unknown causes, and it also exhibits inadequate inter-rater reliability. The proposed method shows potential for clinical application as DL systems continue to develop. Also, the authors of [29] used CNNs on ADC maps to achieve high accuracy to extract features that could assist clinicians in treatment decisions by predicting short-term functional outcomes. However, the decisions were not based on biologically relevant information. To provide localization of regions of interest, an attention-based method was used to examine the CNN's decisions. The final model performed well on both training and validation sets, demonstrating the potential of CNNs to predict short-term functional outcomes accurately.

The severity and location of the brain damage caused by stroke can result in a diverse range of neurological impairment. This can lead to enduring disabilities or even fatality. Although rehabilitation and therapy can ameliorate the patient's quality of life, prompt identification and intervention are crucial to prevent lasting disabilities. In [31] authors built a 3D CNN model to classify neurological impairment caused by ischemic stroke using DWI images, achieving promising results in predicting the NIHSS (National Institutes of Health Stroke Scale) score on Day 7 of hospitalization. By effectively predicting the severity of both anterior and posterior circulation stroke, the model has the potential to assist with clinical decision-making.

Thrombus red blood cell (RBC) content in AIS refers to the amount of RBCs present in the blood clot that obstructs the blood flow to the brain during a stroke. The occurrence of RBCs in the thrombus is a sign of the clot's duration and its capacity to cause additional harm to the brain. High RBC content in the thrombus is associated with worse clinical outcomes in AIS patients, indicating the importance of early recognition and intervention. The [34] study aimed to develop a CNN using multiparametric MRI to predict thrombus RBC content in AIS. The CNN classified MR images of thrombi into RBC-rich and RBC-poor groups with successful results. The accuracy improved with data augmentation techniques, and the CNN could accurately predict thrombus RBC content, potentially guiding treatment strategies in AIS.

Long short-term memory (LSTM) is a type of neural network that can be used to predict stroke functional outcome by modeling the temporal dynamics of clinical features and imaging biomarkers. Using data collected within 24 hours of stroke symptom onset, the model has been utilized to predict the 90-day modified Rankin scale (mRS) score after a stroke. The LSTM model has achieved high accuracy and could help improve stroke patient outcomes. [40] proposes a DL approach for predicting stroke patients' clinical outcome after mechanical thrombectomy. The approach uses a CNN-LSTM ensemble model that considers both clinical metadata and MRI images. The CNN-LSTM is applied autonomously to diffusion and perfusion MRI. The ultimate mRS score is acquired by combining the probabilities of every MRI module, which are weighted by clinical metadata. The approach was successful in achieving an accuracy of 74% and an area under the curve (AUC) of 0.77. However, the current ensemble model is limited to using only one clinical variable, and further research is required to expand the weighting algorithm to integrate multiple clinical variables with multiple image modules. The authors of [42] propose a framework that optimizes deep CNN models like VGG16, ResNet50, and DenseNet121 for efficient detection of brain stroke using MRI scans. The framework uses data augmentation techniques to improve training quality and splits the dataset into training, validation, and testing samples to avoid overfitting. The optimized models significantly improved performance, and an algorithm named ODL-BSD (Optimized Deep Learning for Brain Stroke Detection) was proposed.

4.4 COMPUTED TOMOGRAPHY

A CT scan is a sophisticated medical imaging procedure that utilizes X-rays and state-of-the-art computer technology to generate detailed cross-sectional images of the human body. It is a fast and noninvasive way to detect and diagnose medical conditions such as strokes, injuries, and tumors. A CT scan is faster and more widely available in emergency departments, making it preferable for evaluating strokes due to its ability to detect bleeding in the brain. In contrast, MRI is superior to CT in detecting early or minor strokes and offers more precise imaging of soft tissues, all the while avoiding the use of ionizing radiation on patients. The choice between the two depends on the specific circumstances and the healthcare provider's judgment.

PSO (particle swarm optimization) is a metaheuristic optimization algorithm that is used to solve optimization problems. The goal is to find the best possible solution by optimizing a fitness function that measures the quality of the solution. It has proven to be effective in optimizing various problems across diverse fields including engineering, computer science, and finance. The [14] article proposes using PSO-optimized CNNs to detect stroke in CT brain images. The authors developed a public dataset and evaluated two PSO fine-tuned network architectures (ImageNet & CIFAR-10), achieving close to 99% classification accuracy. They suggest further improving results by augmenting the dataset and trying other DL techniques.

CTP is a type of medical imaging test that uses CT technology to generate detailed images of blood flow in organs and tissues. It provides information about blood flow at a single point in time. On the other hand, 4D CTP (4D CTP) is a type of medical imaging technique that provides detailed information on the blood flow to a specific organ or tissue over time. It uses a series of CT images taken at regular intervals after a contrast dye is injected into the bloodstream to provide information about how blood flow changes over time. In summary, CTP provides information about blood flow at a single point in time, while 4D CTP provides information about blood flow over time.

4.4.1 CT for Lesion

The authors of [20] present a new DL-based method for automatically detecting ischemic stroke lesions using CT perfusion (CTP) data. They use a generative adversarial network (GAN) to generate DWI from CTP data and a CNN with a novel segmentation loss function to segment the stroke lesion on top of the generated DWI. With a four-fold cross-validation technique, the proposed method attains an average dice coefficient of 60.65%, surpassing the performance of conventional methods that rely on CTP perfusion parameters. The authors suggest their pipeline could have potential clinical applications. However,

[30] used 4D CTP scans to forecast the outcomes of AIS directly without using perfusion maps. They developed a new DL model that consists of an encoder, a temporal convolutional network, and a decoder that predicts the probability of infarction at each voxel. The model outperforms perfusion maps and the results show that training on 32 time points is more effective than training on fewer time points. Overall, the model is effective in predicting stroke outcomes from 4D CTP scans.

4.4.2 CT for Stroke

The [6] paper discusses the use of a CNN-based solution for detecting dense vessels and ischemic regions in non-contrast CT scans in AIS cases. The evaluation of a CNN architecture that incorporates contralateral and Anatomical Tracings of Lesions After Stroke (ATLAS) location features indicates that bilateral comparison is essential for the identification of ischemia, and ATLAS location is significant for the detection of dense vessels. The incorporation of ATLAS data is found to be useful for the detection of dense vessels, but not so much for the detection of ischemic regions. In addition, a 3D CNN with kernel spatial decomposition applied one dimension at a time is utilized. It has been determined that the most efficient method is to inject ATLAS data alongside intensity inputs at the input layer. The [39] paper proposes a hybrid approach that uses a novel CNN architecture called OzNet and various ML algorithms to classify brain stroke CT images. By utilizing OzNet as a deep feature extractor and employing a combination of the minimum redundancy maximum relevance (mRMR) technique and classical ML algorithms for feature selection and classification, the study attains an outstanding accuracy level of 87.47%. The hybrid OzNet–mRMR-NB algorithm yields the most optimal outcomes, attaining an accuracy of 98.42% and an AUC of 0.99 when detecting strokes from CT brain images. The study demonstrates the potential of using AI and ML algorithms to improve the detection of neurological disorders, such as stroke. The [22] article describes the development of a two-stage DL model for automatic AIS detection. The model consists of a You Only Look Once v3 (YOLOv3) model for AIS detection and a Visual Geometry Group 16 (VGG16) model for reducing false-positives. The model was tested on 49 cases and compared to a radiologist's evaluation of the same cases, with and without the use of the model's detection results. The findings indicated that the radiologist's detection sensitivity was significantly enhanced by the two-stage model. The research also explores the development of a dataset validated by MRI and CT for assessing AIS detection systems. This [41] study developed a computer-aided diagnosis system using image processing and DL models to detect abnormal areas in brain CTs of stroke patients. A dataset of 1,000 patients was used, and the study demonstrated successful detection and interpretation results using pre-trained DL models. The system could help with early diagnosis of AIS, but doctors' and radiologists' supervision and advice are still necessary. The study's limitations included not having all the CT scan data of every patient.

4.4.3 CT for Early Stroke

The Otsu algorithm is a classic image processing technique that separates an image into foreground and background regions based on intensity values. It finds the optimal threshold that maximizes the variance between the two regions, and can be used in DL for image segmentation tasks or to improve segmentation accuracy. The [5] article describes an automatic system that utilizes a DL CNN algorithm, CT images, and the Otsu algorithm to detect ischemic strokes in their early stages. The system takes small images called patches using different data techniques to increase diversity, and then uses a special type of neural network with layers that help to identify patterns in the data. The neural network has two layers that do convolution, one layer that selects the maximum value, and a final layer that connects all the information together. The system achieved over 90% accuracy in detecting stroke in CT scans and can assist doctors in diagnosing stroke patients quickly and accurately. Future work includes collecting more brain stroke images to improve the system's recognition rate.

4.4.4 CT for Hemorrhagic Stroke

Hemorrhagic stroke develops when a blood vessel in the brain bursts, inducing bleeding and injury to brain tissue. Symptoms include sudden severe headache, numbness, difficulty speaking, vision changes, and loss of coordination. Factors that increase the likelihood of developing hemorrhagic stroke include tobacco use, hypertension, and excessive alcohol consumption. Treatment may involve medications, surgery, and rehabilitation.

[23] proposes a new method for classifying brain CT scan images into hemorrhagic stroke, ischemic stroke, and normal categories using a newly proposed CNN architecture. A new CNN approach was proposed that uses image fusion to extract better features from multiple layers of the network and pre-processing techniques like contrast adjustment and image filtering to enhance CT images. In terms of accuracy, the approach used in the experiments outperformed popular CNN architectures such as AlexNet and ResNet50, as demonstrated in tests conducted on two datasets.

Transfer learning is a technique in DL that uses a pre-trained neural network as a starting point for a new neural network trained on a different task or dataset. By utilizing the learned characteristics of the pre-existing model, it boosts the new model's effectiveness, while simultaneously conserving time and resources. The [37] study suggests a method for automated transfer learning that employs ResNet-50 and a dense layer to achieve precise prediction of intracranial hemorrhage on NCCT brain images. The proposed deep transfer learning approach achieved high accuracy, sensitivity, and specificity in classifying hemorrhagic stroke. The model has potential for use as a clinical decision support tool to assist radiologists in stroke diagnosis. To enhance accuracy and minimize computational complexity, upcoming research will concentrate on utilizing various transfer learning approaches to classify subtypes and locate intracerebral hemorrhage (ICH) lesions.

4.4.5 CT for Others

The [17] article explores the use of DL methods for predicting stroke outcomes using CT angiography images. The model demonstrates superior performance compared to conventional radiological image biomarkers, and does not necessitate image annotation, while also being fast. However, the predictive value is still relatively low, and future models should incorporate clinical characteristics. Model visualization tools are used to improve interpretability.

Infarct volume refers to the amount of tissue in the brain that has died or become damaged as a result of reduced blood flow, typically caused by a stroke or other similar conditions. It is measured in cubic centimeters (cc) or milliliters (ml) using medical imaging techniques such as CT or MRI scans. The infarct volume can help doctors assess the severity of the damage, predict the patient's recovery, and determine the most appropriate treatment plan. [24] aims to assess the effectiveness of a CNN in anticipating the extent of infarction based on CTA images in patients experiencing anterior circulation ischemic stroke. The CNN model proved effective in detecting acute ischemic lesions and providing accurate estimates of infarct core volumes. The infarct volumes obtained from the CNN were compared with CTP-RAPID ischemic core volumes and final infarct volumes measured from follow-up CT images. While the infarct volumes obtained from the CNN exhibited a strong correlation with the final infarct volumes, the correlation between the CTP-RAPID and final infarct volumes was even more substantial. The study concluded that the CNN model can be a useful tool in stroke diagnosis and treatment decision-making.

Long-term functional outcome in stroke refers to the degree of disability or impairment that a patient experiences following a stroke, and how well they are able to function in their daily life in the months and years following the event. Impairments, which can impact an individual's capacity to engage in social interactions, perform daily activities, and pursue hobbies or work of personal significance, may encompass cognitive, emotional, and physical limitations. Long-term functional outcome is an important factor in stroke prognosis and treatment planning, and can be influenced by a variety of factors, including the type and severity of the stroke, the timing and effectiveness of treatment, and the patient's overall health and wellbeing. The [32] research employed a CNN-based DL model to forecast long-term functional results in patients who suffered from ischemic stroke, utilizing DWI taken on the first day following the stroke. The CNN model was better than other methods at predicting poor outcomes, defined as mRS>2 three months after a stroke. By using an attention mechanism, the network learned to focus on the lesion when predicting outcomes. This study proposes that hospitals could use the CNN model to enhance patient care and outcomes.

4.5 OTHER THAN CT & MRI IMAGING MODALITIES

Other than CT and MRI we can use data in order to diagnose brain disorders like biomarkers (ECG, electroencephalogram (EEG) [26], electromyography (EMG), electrooculography (EOG), retinal fundus images [28, 36]). And also instead of images (CT or CTP), structured data can also be used as in [33].

4.5.1 For Stroke Diagnosis

EEG – It evaluates the brain's electrical patterns and can be utilized for the diagnosis and monitoring of neurological disorders like epilepsy, sleep disorders, and brain injuries. It is also used in research to study brain activity during different tasks or in response to stimuli. EEG is safe and painless, and typically takes 30 to 60 minutes to complete. The resulting

EEG signal can be analyzed to detect abnormalities or changes in brain function. In the [26] paper, a stroke prediction model is suggested that utilizes EEG data obtained from sensors in real time. The model accomplished 94% accuracy while also keeping false-positive and false-negative rates low. This model can detect stroke risk promptly, enabling access to treatment within the critical period. However, authors of [28] propose a model for automated stroke diagnosis using retinal fundus images. The authors compared hand-crafted features with DL approaches and concluded that the custom CNN model is superior in accuracy. The study highlights the potential of DL in healthcare and bioinformatics fields for disease detection.

Instead of 2D or 3D CNN we can use 1D CNN if data is sequential. The paper [33] uses 1D CNN and features selection methods to extract structured features, achieving an accuracy of 95.5%. [33] presents a CNN model for predicting stroke in patients using a healthcare dataset with 11 features. The study also analyzed the correlation between stroke risk and various factors, showing that age, BMI, and average glucose level were highly associated with stroke risk. The proposed model shows promise in predicting stroke disease and can be applied in clinical settings.

4.5.2 For Early Stroke Prediction

The authors of [36] propose a framework that uses DL techniques like LSTM, biLSTM, GRU, and Gated Recurrent Unit and Feed Forward Neural Networks (FFNN) to predict strokes using EEG signals. The experimental results show that GRU outperforms others with an accuracy of 95.6%. The framework is noninvasive, quick, and can make predictions on online data for early detection of strokes. It can assist physicians in starting quick treatments for stroke prevention.

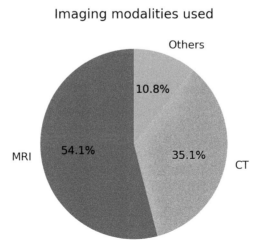

FIGURE 4.2   Pie chart for percentage of different imaging modalities used in the papers we have reviewed.

4.6 LIMITATIONS & FUTURE TRENDS

The number of papers reviewed is less (44) and are mostly from year 2022 (refer Figure 4.1); papers are not equally distributed year-wise. The papers mostly focus on imaging modalities and DL models. In future we might go for more papers with different imaging modalities and models.

4.7 CONCLUSION

Here in this review we have discussed various DL models for various stroke conditions. Though various models are being developed for various imaging modalities (Figure 4.2), there is still need for many more different and effective DL models for easy and cost-effective imaging modalities like CT, so that all patients can benefit. Also, there are models that make use of biomarkers for efficient diagnosis of stroke like EEG, retinal fundus images, which is what we have discussed in Section 4.5.

REFERENCES

[1] Stier, N., Vincent, N., Liebeskind, D., & Scalzo, F. (2015, November). Deep learning of tissue fate features in acute ischemic stroke. In *2015 IEEE International Conference on Bioinformatics and Biomedicine (BIBM)* (pp. 1316–1321). IEEE.

[2] Choi, Y., Kwon, Y., Lee, H., Kim, B. J., Paik, M. C., & Won, J. H. (2016). Ensemble of deep convolutional neural networks for prognosis of ischemic stroke. In *Brainlesion: Glioma, Multiple Sclerosis, Stroke and Traumatic Brain Injuries: Second International Workshop, BrainLes 2016, with the Challenges on BRATS, ISLES and mTOP 2016*, Held in Conjunction with MICCAI 2016, Athens, Greece, October 17, 2016, Revised Selected Papers 2 (pp. 231–243). Springer International Publishing.

[3] Kamnitsas, K., Ledig, C., Newcombe, V. F., Simpson, J. P., Kane, A. D., Menon, D. K., ... & Glocker, B. (2017). Efficient multi-scale 3D CNN with fully connected CRF for accurate brain lesion segmentation. *Medical Image Analysis*, 36, 61–78.

[4] Lee, E. J., Kim, Y. H., Kim, N., & Kang, D. W. (2017). Deep into the brain: Artificial intelligence in stroke imaging. *Journal of Stroke*, 19(3), 277–285.

[5] Chin, C. L., Lin, B. J., Wu, G. R., Weng, T. C., Yang, C. S., Su, R. C., & Pan, Y. J. (2017, November). An automated early ischemic stroke detection system using CNN deep learning algorithm. In *2017 IEEE 8th International Conference on Awareness Science and Technology (iCAST)* (pp. 368–372). IEEE.

[6] Lisowska, A., O'Neil, A., Dilys, V., Daykin, M., Beveridge, E., Muir, K., ... & Poole, I. (2017). Context-aware convolutional neural networks for stroke sign detection in non-contrast CT scans. In *Medical Image Understanding and Analysis: 21st Annual Conference, MIUA 2017*, Edinburgh, UK, July 11–13, 2017, Proceedings 21 (pp. 494–505). Springer International Publishing.

[7] Akkus, Z., Galimzianova, A., Hoogi, A., Rubin, D. L., & Erickson, B. J. (2017). Deep learning for brain MRI segmentation: State of the art and future directions. *Journal of Digital Imaging*, 30, 449–459.

[8] Chen, L., Bentley, P., & Rueckert, D. (2017). Fully automatic acute ischemic lesion segmentation in DWI using convolutional neural networks. *NeuroImage: Clinical*, 15, 633–643.

[9] Jiang, F., Jiang, Y., Zhi, H., Dong, Y., Li, H., Ma, S., ... & Wang, Y. (2017). Artificial intelligence in healthcare: Past, present and future. *Stroke and Vascular Neurology*, 2(4), 230–243.

[10] Feng, R., Badgeley, M., Mocco, J., & Oermann, E. K. (2018). Deep learning guided stroke management: A review of clinical applications. *Journal of Neurointerventional Surgery*, 10(4), 358–362.

[11] Nielsen, A., Hansen, M. B., Tietze, A., & Mouridsen, K. (2018). Prediction of tissue outcome and assessment of treatment effect in acute ischemic stroke using deep learning. *Stroke*, 49(6), 1394–1401.

[12] Liew, S. L., Anglin, J. M., Banks, N. W., Sondag, M., Ito, K. L., Kim, H., ... & Stroud, A. (2018). A large, open source dataset of stroke anatomical brain images and manual lesion segmentations. *Scientific Data*, 5(1), 1–11.

[13] Winzeck, S., Hakim, A., McKinley, R., Pinto, J. A., Alves, V., Silva, C., ... & Reyes, M. (2018). ISLES 2016 and 2017-benchmarking ischemic stroke lesion outcome prediction based on multispectral MRI. *Frontiers in Neurology*, 9, 679.

[14] Pereira, D. R., ReboucasFilho, P. P., de Rosa, G. H., Papa, J. P., & de Albuquerque, V. H. C. (2018, July). Stroke lesion detection using convolutional neural networks. In *2018 International Joint Conference on Neural Networks (IJCNN)* (pp. 1–6). IEEE.

[15] Chauhan, S., Vig, L., De Filippo De Grazia, M., Corbetta, M., Ahmad, S., & Zorzi, M. (2019). A comparison of shallow and deep learning methods for predicting cognitive performance of stroke patients from MRI lesion images. *Frontiers in Neuroinformatics*, 13, 53.

[16] Zhu, G., Jiang, B., Tong, L., Xie, Y., Zaharchuk, G., & Wintermark, M. (2019). Applications of deep learning to neuro-imaging techniques. *Frontiers in Neurology*, 10, 869.

[17] Hilbert, A., Ramos, L. A., van Os, H. J., Olabarriaga, S. D., Tolhuisen, M. L., Wermer, M. J., ... & Marquering, H. A. (2019). Data-efficient deep learning of radiological image data for outcome prediction after endovascular treatment of patients with acute ischemic stroke. *Computers in Biology and Medicine*, 115, 103516.

[18] Meier, R., Lux, P., Jung, S., Fischer, U., Gralla, J., Reyes, M., ... & Kaesmacher, J. (2019). Neural network–derived perfusion maps for the assessment of lesions in patients with acute ischemic stroke. *Radiology: Artificial Intelligence*, 1(5), e190019.

[19] Perez Malla, C. U., Valdes Hernandez, M. D. C., Rachmadi, M. F., & Komura, T. (2019). Evaluation of enhanced learning techniques for segmenting ischaemic stroke lesions in brain magnetic resonance perfusion images using a convolutional neural network scheme. *Frontiers in Neuroinformatics*, 13, 33.

[20] Liu, P. (2019). Stroke lesion segmentation with 2D novel CNN pipeline and novel loss function. In *Brainlesion: Glioma, Multiple Sclerosis, Stroke and Traumatic Brain Injuries: 4th International Workshop, BrainLes 2018*, Held in Conjunction with MICCAI 2018, Granada, Spain, September 16, 2018, Revised Selected Papers, Part I 4 (pp. 253–262). Springer International Publishing.

[21] Sathish, R., Rajan, R., Vupputuri, A., Ghosh, N., & Sheet, D. (2019, July). Adversarially trained convolutional neural networks for semantic segmentation of ischaemic stroke lesion using multisequence magnetic resonance imaging. In *2019 41st Annual International Conference of the IEEE Engineering in Medicine and Biology Society (EMBC)* (pp. 1010–1013). IEEE.

[22] Nishio, M., Koyasu, S., Noguchi, S., Kiguchi, T., Nakatsu, K., Akasaka, T., ... & Itoh, K. (2020). Automatic detection of acute ischemic stroke using non-contrast computed tomography and two- stage deep learning model. *Computer Methods and Programs in Biomedicine*, 196, 105711.

[23] Gautam, A., & Raman, B. (2021). Towards effective classification of brain hemorrhagic and ischemic stroke using CNN. *Biomedical Signal Processing and Control*, 63, 102178.

[24] Hokkinen, L., Mäkelä, T., Savolainen, S., & Kangasniemi, M. (2021). Evaluation of a CTA-based convolutional neural network for infarct volume prediction in anterior cerebral circulation ischaemic stroke. *European Radiology Experimental*, 5, 1–11.

[25] Zhang, S., Xu, S., Tan, L., Wang, H., & Meng, J. (2021). Stroke lesion detection and analysis in MRI images based on deep learning. *Journal of Healthcare Engineering*, 2021, 1–9.

[26] Choi, Y. A., Park, S. J., Jun, J. A., Pyo, C. S., Cho, K. H., Lee, H. S., & Yu, J. H. (2021). Deep learning-based stroke disease prediction system using real-time bio signals. *Sensors*, 21(13), 4269.

[27] Park, S., Kim, B. K., Han, M. K., Hong, J. H., Yum, K. S., & Lee, D. I. (2021). Deep learning for prediction of mechanism in acute ischemic stroke using brain MRI. Retrieved from https://doi.org/10.21203/rs.3.rs-604141/v1

[28] Jeena, R. S., Shiny, G., Sukesh Kumar, A., & Mahadevan, K. (2021). A comparative analysis of stroke diagnosis from retinal images using hand-crafted features and CNN. *Journal of Intelligent & Fuzzy Systems*, 41(5), 5327–5335.

[29] Zihni, E., McGarry, B. L., & Kelleher, J. D. (2021). An analysis of the interpretability of neural networks trained on magnetic resonance imaging for stroke outcome prediction. *Proceedings of the International Society for Magnetic Resonance in Medicine*, 29, 3503.

[30] Amador, K., Wilms, M., Winder, A., Fiehler, J., & Forkert, N. (2021, August). Stroke lesion outcome prediction based on 4d CT perfusion data using temporal convolutional networks. In *Medical Imaging with Deep Learning*, 22–33. PMLR.

[31] Zeng, Y., Long, C., Zhao, W., & Liu, J. (2022). Predicting the severity of neurological impairment caused by ischemic stroke using deep learning based on diffusion-weighted images. *Journal of Clinical Medicine*, 11(14), 4008.

[32] Moulton, E., Valabregue, R., Piotin, M., Marnat, G., Saleme, S., Lapergue, B., … & Rosso, C. (2023). Interpretable deep learning for the prognosis of long-term functional outcome post-stroke using acute diffusion weighted imaging. *Journal of Cerebral Blood Flow & Metabolism*, 43(2), 198–209.

[33] Ashrafuzzaman, M., Saha, S., & Nur, K. (2022). Prediction of stroke disease using deep CNN Based approach. *Journal of Advances in Information Technology*, 13(6), 604–613.

[34] Christiansen, S. D., Liu, J., Bullrich, M. B., Sharma, M., Boulton, M., Pandey, S. K., Sposato, L. A. & Drangova, M. (2022). Deep learning prediction of stroke thrombus red blood cell content from multiparametric MRI. *Interventional Neuroradiology*. https://doi.org/10.1177/15910199221140962.

[35] Alotaibi, N. S., Alotaibi, A. S., Eliazer, M., & Srinivasulu, A. (2022). Detection of ischemic stroke tissue fate from the MRI images using a deep learning approach. *Mobile Information Systems*, Article ID 9399876. https://doi.org/10.1155/2022/9399876.

[36] Kaur, M., Sakhare, S. R., Wanjale, K., & Akter, F. (2022). Early stroke prediction methods for prevention of strokes. *Behavioural Neurology*, Article ID 7725597. https://doi.org/10.1155/2022/7725597.

[37] Rao, B. N., Mohanty, S., Sen, K., Acharya, U. R., Cheong, K. H., & Sabut, S. (2022). Deep transfer learning for automatic prediction of hemorrhagic stroke on CT images. *Computational and Mathematical Methods in Medicine*, https://doi.org/10.1155/2022/3560507.

[38] Soun, J. E., Chow, D. S., Nagamine, M., Takhtawala, R. S., Filippi, C. G., Yu, W., & Chang, P. D. (2021). Artificial intelligence and acute stroke imaging. *American Journal of Neuroradiology*, 42(1), 2–11.

[39] Ozaltin, O., Coskun, O., Yeniay, O., & Subasi, A. (2022). A deep learning approach for detecting stroke from brain CT images using oznet. *Bioengineering*, 9(12), 783.

[40] Hatami, N., Cho, T. H., Mechtouff, L., Eker, O. F., Rousseau, D., & Frindel, C. (2022). CNN-LSTM based multimodal MRI and clinical data fusion for predicting functional outcome in stroke patients. arXiv preprint arXiv:2205.05545.

[41] URAL, A. B. (2022). Computer aided deep learning based assessment of stroke from brain radiological CT images. *Avrupa Bilimve Teknoloji Dergisi*, (34), 42–52. https://doi.org/10.31590/ejosat.1063356.

[42] Kashi Sai Prasad, D. R. (2022). Deep convolutional neural network implementations for efficient brain stroke detection using MRI scans. *Journal of Theoretical and Applied Information Technology*, 100(17), 5467–5481.

[43] Nugroho, A. K., Putranto, T. A., Purnama, I. K. E., & Purnomo, M. H. Quad Convolutional Layers (QCL) CNN Approach for classification of brain stroke in Diffusion Weighted (DW)-Magnetic Resonance Images (MRI). International Journal of Intelligent Engineering & Systems, 15(1), https://doi.org/10.22266/ijies2022.0228.38.

CHAPTER 5

A Framework for Brain Tumor Image Compression with Principal Component Analysis

Application of Machine Learning in Neuroimaging

Subhagata Chattopadhyay

5.1 INTRODUCTION

Brain tumors (BRTs) are devastating due to the high mortality rate and poor quality of life after survival. It hardly matters whether it is cancerous or not. The 'mass or pressure effect' of the unregulated growth of the neural cells compresses the adjacent areas of the brain tissue, its vascular supply, thus disturbing the electromechanical activities and its coordination. Cancerous growth is much more aggressive and kills faster than benign growth. It is important to note that one-third of BRTs are cancerous (Cleveland Clinic, 2022). The International Association of Cancer Registers shows about 28,000 such cases in India and 24,000 die annually as reported by an esteemed Indian daily (The Hindu, 2021). Headache of various types, intractable vomiting, neck rigidity, fits, vision changes, behavioral dysregulations, partial or total loss of consciousness, and sometimes absolutely silence are some of the key signs of BRT. About 5% BRTs are hereditary (John Hopkins Medicine, 2022). BRTs that originate in the brain itself are called primary tumors and those coming from the other parts of the body are known as metastatic tumors. The latter is more virulent than the former. Hence, the earlier it is screened, the better the prognosis.

The *origin* of primary BRTs is from the brain itself or the adjacent tissues when the DNA is mutated inside the cells of origin and increases the ratio of an oncogene (a gene that produces more and more cells) and tumor suppressor gene (a gene that suppresses

DOI: 10.1201/9781003264767-5

the production of an excessive number of cells). Cancers are caused when the tumor suppressor genes are turned off and oncogenes are turned on causing an unopposed relentless growth of brain cells (American Cancer Society, 2020). The stem, progenitor, and differentiated cell types are tumorigenic (Azzarelli, Simons, & Philpott, 2018). CD15- and CD133-positive cells are potentially tumorigenic (Azzarelli, Simons, & Philpott, 2018). Among many causative agents, radiation, exposure to an electromagnetic field, HIV infection, and cell phones fall on the non-exhaustive list (American Cancer Society, 2020).

The *investigational modalities* of BRTs are essentially radiological and bestowed on computerized tomography (CT) and magnetic resonance imaging (MRI) scans. A study has reported that around 9.2 lacs of CT and 80,000 MRI scans are performed in India annually for diagnosis and assessing the prognosis of the condition and more importantly its numbers are growing (Narayan, 2019). A CT takes pictures of the brain from various angles using an X-ray and with the help of the computer, these are combined into a 3D image. It can measure the size of the tumor. A dye-guided CT is performed to get a picture of the vasculature in and around the tumor. CT is indicated when the patient has a pacemaker as an MRI scan which may interfere with the pacemaker function, and it is contraindicated here. A CT is also cheaper than MRI scans. Although the latter is the preferred method for detecting BRTs, image size, shape, and extension are more clear as compared to a CT.

MRI and CT images are usually of larger pixel sizes when compared to X-rays. The number of CT and MRI scans is exponentially increasing due to their reduced cost and given that it is the key diagnostic modality in the neurosciences. To handle it faster without losing much of the data, the application of the image compression technique using *principal component analysis (PCA)* is a popular statistical machine learning (ML) technique at the outset of medical image processing to reduce its size by discarding correlated variables/features (called 'observed variable data space'), preserving information of non-correlated variables of higher multi-dimensional space to lower-dimensional subspace, which is called as the 'independent variable data space' (Nandi, Ashour, Samanta, Chakraborty, & Abdel-Megeed Mohammed Salem, 2015; Roopa & Asha, 2018). Hence, PCA provides efficient information management as well as dimensionality reductions and can extract non-correlated features from an image (Taur & Tao, 1996). The importance of PCA has become multi-fold due to the gain in automatic detection of anomalies, abnormalities, and several pathological conditions in medical image processing (Bhandary et al., 2020).

In the present work, the author has addressed the *research question* of how to proficiently reduce the BRT image sizes for increasing the efficiency of an automated tool to screen BRTs. PCA has been used to compress BRT images to study how efficiently it can compress the images with much loss of image clarity through graded parametric studies. *Image quality assessment (IQA)* has been performed for each of the compressed images to examine the performance of PCA, For assessing image quality, the mean quality score (MQS) of the compressed images is measured, which is followed by examining *computational complexity (Big(O))* of the algorithms used in this work.

5.2 LITERATURE REVIEW

PCA, also popularly known as *Hotelling Transform* or *Karhunen-Loeve Transform*, is a statistical ML technique, used principally for dimensionality reduction of a large dataset. Originally it was proposed by Karl Pearson in 1901 as part of factorial analysis (Pearson, 1901). The development happened in 1933 by Hotelling (1933) (Jackson, 1991; Jolliffe, 2002; Wichern & Johnson, 2014). Delay in the development of the PCA algorithm had happened due to the lack of computer facilities at that time (Diamantaras & Kung, 1996). Image datasets are inherently large and hence PCA remains one of the gold standard statistical ML techniques for image processing (Mohammed, Khalid, Osman, & Helali, 2016). There are several studies reported to date where PCA has been used for (i) image compression (Yang et al., 2017), (ii) image segmentation (Mao et al., 2019), (iii) feature extraction (Wang et al., 2016), (iv) image fusion (Metwalli, Nasr, Farag Allah, & El-Rabaie, 2009), (v) image denoising/cleaning (Ai, Yang, Fan, Cong, & Wang, 2015), and (vi) image registration (Nandi, Ashour, Samanta, Chakraborty, & Abdel-Megeed Mohammed Salem, 2015). Some important studies (but not an exhaustive list) have been discussed below in a nutshell where PCA has been used for several purposes.

Dimensionality reduction of images is an important preliminary step not only to reduce the computational complexity but also in extracting principal components, which can be further utilized to train a classifier for more efficiency in terms of speed and accuracy by enhancing the learning process. A group of researchers studied PCA-mined chest X-ray (CXR) image information for the diagnosis of COVID19 using convolutional neural network (CNN) and logistic regression (LR) (Rasheed, Ali Hameed, Djeddi, Jamil, & Al-Turjman, 2021). To overcome the issue of data overfitting, the authors used a generative adversarial network (GAN). A total of 500 CXRs have been studied. The study concludes that LR and CNN models can diagnose COVID19 cases with 95.2%–97.6% total accuracy without the application of PCA. With PCA application, the accuracy increases by 97.6%–100%.

PCA has been used to reduce dimension as a measure of image data preprocessing in images showing bony fractures. The aim is to classify fractures automatically without any loss of data reliability, which is important for accurate classification (Doorsamy & Rameshar, 2021). The authors used ANFIS, ANN, and SVM (support vector machine) classifiers. The study concludes that with an appreciable level of compression (up to 94%), the classification accuracy drops only by 2%, which means that PCA can maintain the originality of the data by as good as 98%.

Performances of wavelet difference reduction (WDR) and PCA have been compared in an extensive study conducted on CT scan images of the lower abdomen and X-ray images of the rib cage (Saradha Rani, Sasibhushana Rao, & Prabhakara Rao, 2019). The study observed that PCA is more efficient in reducing image dimensionality, while WDR is a better tool for image reconstruction without much data loss.

PCA and kernel PCA (kPCA) are used to analyze the extracted features of CXRs showing pulmonary tuberculosis with efficient compression of the higher dimensionality (Roopa & Asha, 2018). Filter and wrapper techniques are used to achieve the desired compression. The compressed features are then passed through a linear regressions classifier for diagnosis. Results show that PCA using the wrapper method provides better accuracy of 96.07%, compared to kPCA using the filter method, which gives an accuracy of 62.50%.

In another interesting study, the performance of PCA was studied on 250 color images to see the critical reduction of the number of features/components due to dimensionality reduction by PCA that produces 'lossy' images and thus increases mean squared error (MSE) and peak signal-to-noise ratio (PSNR) (Abbas, Arab, & Harbi, 2018). The authors state that the reasons behind such occurrence are (i) converting color image to grayscale image, where considerable data is lost, and (ii) converting all pixel values in a vector and determining the best eigenvectors associated with the maximum of the eigenvalues, leaving other eigenvectors in place.

Efficient image compression using PCA mingled with Linear Algebra has been studied by Hernandez & Mendez (2018). The authors used this hybrid method (several PCA methods plus lemmas of Linear Algebra) for reconstructing good-quality images post-compression. To reduce the computational cost, a novel construction of principal components by using the periodicity of principal components was introduced in the study, although the accuracy level was compromised. The study finally concluded that using almost all periodicity of the first principal component, acceptable quality of reconstructed images can be obtained with less information loss.

PCA has been efficiently used for content-based image retrieval from the image Picture Archiving and Communication System (PACS) database (Sinha & Kangarloo, 2002). The key reason behind such an encouraging result is that PCA produced prototype images by reducing the original dimensionality but preserving the original data veracity, which helps the search algorithm to find out the desired images. It has been applied to 100 axial brain images from a 3D T1-weighted MRI study. The algorithm has been evaluated by using 96 axial images from eight patients. The study concludes that PCA can help search and retrieve the target image from the large electronic database, based on the high-quality prototype images it can produce.

Above, some benchmarked published literature has been reviewed. As mentioned before, this is not an exhaustive list and all the literature cannot be cited due to space constraints. However, summarily, it can be noted how useful PCA can be in today's automation in medical image processing.

5.2.1 The gap in the Literature and Contribution of the Current Work

The efficiency of PCA has been traded off between level (%) of compression and loss of data veracity during preprocessing-to-classification tasks. However, no study has been reported so far on determining the *critical number* of components and validating it 'quantitatively' on plain CXRs of both genders. It would assist the researchers to design and develop classifiers for CXR analysis in determining the 'critical' number of components with which prototype images can be well reconstructed without much loss of 'clarity'. In this study, the author has addressed this gap by examining the effective compression % vs. image quality thus obtained by computing MQS as an IQA technique for the compressed CXR images of both males and females.

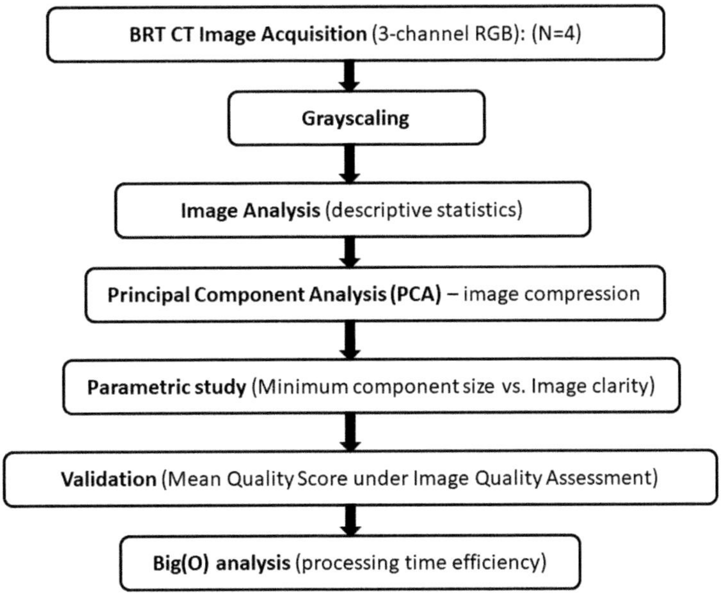

FIGURE 5.1 Flow diagram of the methodology.

It is worth noting that throughout the study the BRTs are coined as 'lesions' irrespective of their types. This chapter does not intend to diagnose the types of BRTs. Its aim is to describe a methodology for image compression optimally.

In the next section, the material and methods for the proposed work have been described step by step. Figure 5.1 shows the methods and techniques used in this study as a flow diagram.

5.3 METHODOLOGY

In this section, the methodology of the study has been discussed step by step as follows. At the outset, details of the programming language and operating system (OS) information have been given, followed by image acquisition and image processing steps.

5.3.1 Programming Language and the OS

Python 3.8.3 with Spyder editor version 4.1.5 was preloaded with *matplotlib, skimage, numpy,* and *sklearn.* All simulations were primarily run on *Windows 10 Pro 64 bits OS x 64-based Processor Intel(R) Core TM @ 2.80 GHz.*

5.3.2 BRT Image Acquisition

To execute the study, with the keyword 'brain tumor images copyright free' in google search four images of a CT brain with lesions are downloaded. Precautions have been taken to check whether these images are 'copyright free' (Figure 5.2).

Source URL: *https://www.google.com/search?q=brain+tumor+photos+copyright+free&source=lnms&tbm=isch&sa=X&ved=2ahUKEwjB2cKLy8P4AhU1-DgGHZklAvcQ_AUoAXoECAEQAw&biw=1517&bih=694&dpr=0.9*

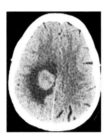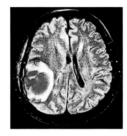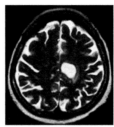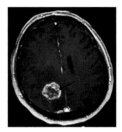

FIGURE 5.2   Original CT images (RGB) of lesions.

5.3.3 Image Processing

The shape and number of features of these images can be seen in Table 5.1. Descriptive statistics of the features are obtained for four grayscaled CT images to obtain data distributions as the maximum, minimum, mean, standard deviations, and quartile distributions for both the features and their values.

PCA has then been performed to extract the minimum number of critical components (i.e., for dimensionality reduction without much loss of original pixel data), with which the prototype images are reconstructed. After the minimum number of components is obtained, its number is increased in a graded fashion (parametric study) to obtain the best clarity keeping the number of components minimum, i.e., higher image compression %. Afterward, using the *BEISQUE algorithm*, the *MQS* is calculated for all images to corroborate the desired output that with the minimum number of components (i.e., higher compression); still higher-quality images can be obtained in a measured fashion and just not subjective visual perception. Finally, *Big(O)* is computed for processing time complexity on various component sizes. These are explained below in detail.

5.3.4 Preprocessing

Step 1: .jpg to.png conversion to obtain 'lossless Raster image'

Step 2: .png to grayscaling to convert three-channel RGB pixels into one-channel Global Shutter (GS) pixels (refer to Figure 5.3)

Step 3: data scaling

Step 4: computing data shape after scaling

Step 5: extracting the shape of the image as rows (height) by columns (weight) and total features by multiplying the number of rows and columns

5.3.5 Descriptive Statistics of Sample Male and Female CXRs

Step 6: descriptive statistics gives the feel of data in an image. Table 5.1 shows the descriptive statistics of the BRT images

5.3.6 PCA

Step 7: fitting scaled data into PCA model

Step 8: computing cumulative variance of pixels

Step 9: computing minimum number of components explaining 95% pixel variance

Step 10: scree plotting to visualize the result of Step 8

Step 11: reconstructing prototype image with minimum parameters/components (*parametric study*) and seeing its quality, i.e., image clarity

Step 12: visualization of the image series *reconstructed* from different sizes of the components

5.3.7 Image Quality Assessment

Step 13: IQA is an important step to validate the quality of the prototype images, reconstructed by PCA after compression. Visually IQA is a subjective task. There are three types of IQAs – (i) *full reference*, where, a seemingly 'distorted' image is compared to a relatively 'clean' version of the same image, (ii) *reduced reference* – here the test image is compared against the similar image with some selective information (e.g., watermarked image), and (iii) *no reference* – in this case, there is no reference image to compare (Ocampo, 2019). In this work, it is presumed that none of the acquired images are of high quality as these essentially are secondary; therefore '*No reference IQA*' has been considered and the name of the algorithm used is BLIND/ REFERENCELESS IMAGE SPATIAL QUALITY EVALUATOR, in short popularly known as BRISQUE (Shrimali, 2018). It depends on the Natural Scene Statistics (NSS) model (refer to equation 5.4) of locally normalized luminance coefficients in the spatial domain and also the model for pairwise products of these coefficients (Shrimali, 2018). Here, the MQS is computed for each image using BRISQUE (with *inequality.brisque* function in Python) using equations 5.1–5.3. The value of MQS varies between 0 and 100, where values closer to 0 indicate a better quality image and vice versa (Shrimali, 2018). In this study gain in MQS (*MQS_gain*) has been computed by comparing the MQS of the minimum component to MQS value of the compressed component size with which qualities almost similar to the original images are obtained (detailed results can be seen in Table 5.2)

$$IM(i,j) = \frac{I(i,j) - \mu(i,j)}{\sigma(i.j) + c} \tag{5.1}$$

In this equation I(I,j), μ(I,j), 'c', and $\sigma(i.j)$ are Image(pixel size), local mean subtraction (see equation 5.2), constant, and local deviation (see equation 5.3), respectively, using which locally normalized luminescence (IM(I,j)) has been computed.

$$\mu(i,j) = \sum_{k=-K}^{K} \sum_{l=-L}^{L} w_{k,l} I_{k,l}(i,j) \tag{5.2}$$

$$\sigma(i.j) = \sqrt{\sum_{k=-K}^{K} \sum_{l=-L}^{L} w_{k,l} \left(I_{k,l}(i,j) \right) - \mu(i,j)} \qquad (5.3)$$

5.3.8 Calculation of Computational Complexity (Big(O))

It is calculated as the number of pixels viewed several times. In all images, each pixel is viewed two times – vertically and horizontally (Schellekens, 2019). Hence, the computational complexity would be

$$Big(O) = (2n) \qquad (5.4)$$

In equation 5.4, 'n' refers to the pixel number. Figure 5.6 plots Big(O) vs. component size for a clearer understanding.

5.4 RESULTS AND DISCUSSION

5.4.1 BRT Images

The covariance matrix shape of the BRT images is (181, 191), (111, 138), (139, 151), and (216, 234). The covariance matrix is an important measure that provides a useful clue for separating the structured relationships in a matrix of random variables (here, pixels). It decorrelates the variables in the matrix dimension. It is the key parameter used in PCA for dimensionality reduction. A positive covariance indicates a strong relationship between any two variables and vice versa. In this work, image compression is conducted with a minimum number of components that can explain 95% of total variances, which means that the information loss would be permitted only up to 5%, which is minimal. Figure 5.3 shows the grayscaled version of the RGB images.

5.4.2 Descriptive Statistics

Descriptive statistics measures see how the features and their corresponding values are distributed and whether these are comparable. Table 5.1 shows the descriptive statistics of the BRT images. Here, it can be noted that the mean feature values (Feature_val) of the sample BRT images are closely comparable. The average comparability is *68%*.

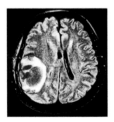 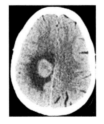 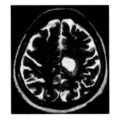 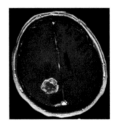

FIGURE 5.3   Grayscaled BRT images.

TABLE 5.1   Descriptive statistics of four BRT images

Parameter	Feature_size				Feature_val			
	1	2	3	4	1	2	3	4
Count	34571	15318	20989	50544	34571	15318	20989	50544
Mean	17285	7658.5	10494	25271.5	0.301683	0.510081	0.256408	0.226398
Std	9979.93	4422.07	6059.147	14590.94	0.273649	0.317472	0.220266	0.183499
Min	0	0	0	0	0	0	0	0
25%	8642.5	3829.25	5247	12635.75	0.013171	0.376471	0.047059	0.015686
50%	17285	7658.5	10494	25271.5	0.296992	0.545098	0.235294	0.258824
75%	25927.5	11487.75	15741	37907.25	0.535419	0.670588	0.337255	0.309804
Max	34570	15317	20988	50543	1	1	1	1

5.4.3 Histogram of Grayscaled Images

Grayscaled value distribution showing the frequency of occurrence of each gray-level value can be seen in an image histogram. In other words, it is a plot of pixel intensity values and their corresponding frequency of occurrence (Vij & Singh, 2011). Its X-axis shows the pixel intensity (brightness) and the corresponding number of pixels (frequency), which are plotted along the Y-axis. This explains that all available gray levels are across the X-axis, while that particular gray-level value can be seen along the Y-axis. The left side of the X-axis refers to darker pixels ('1' denotes the perfect dark) while the right side of it refers to shadows or brighter pixels ('0' denotes the brightest pixel). The middle portion ('0.5') refers to the exact mid-tone. Figure 5.4 shows the histogram plots.

It is noted that maximum pixel values fall in the mid-tone areas. Based on these parameters, histograms can be used for image thresholding.

5.4.4 PCA Results

As mentioned above, using the covariance information, PCA has been conducted on CT BRT images and plotted (scree plot). It plots the number of components along the X-axis vs. cumulative explained variance along the Y-axis. It can be noted that images 1 to 4 can be represented by 39, 16, 26, and 35 components. Each of these component sizes can explain 95% of the cumulative variance. Hence, the images can be compressed by 39/191, i.e., 80%; 16/138, i.e., 88%; 26/151, i.e., 83%; and 35/234, i.e., 85%, respectively, with an average compression of 84%, which are quite appreciable results. Figure 5.5a through d show the scree plots and the respective images in the same rack.

5.4.5 Image Reconstruction (Parametric Study)

With minimum components, the clarities of the prototype CT BRT image samples, which are reconstructed images, are found to be relatively poor or 'lossy', when compared to

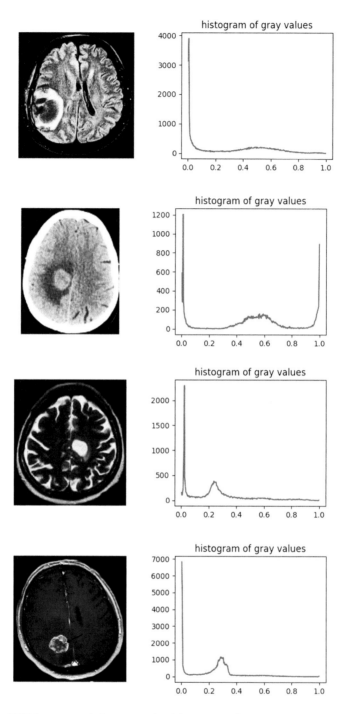

FIGURE 5.4   The BRT images and the respective histogram plots.

original (control) images. To increase the clarity (i.e., decrease the loss-ness) of the compressed images, the sizes of the components are parametrized in a graded fashion starting from the average number of components, where 29 represents 95% covariance in the images. Figure 5.6 shows the prototype reconstructed images with component sizes ranging from 26 (compression level: 84%) to double the size, i.e., 52 (compression level: 70%).

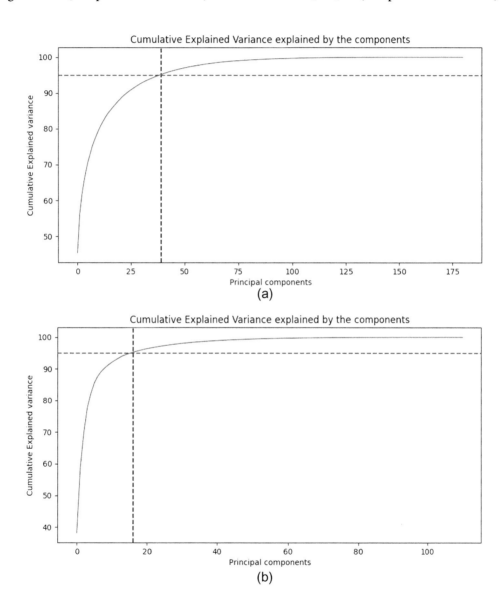

FIGURE 5.5   Scree plots of the CT BRT images.

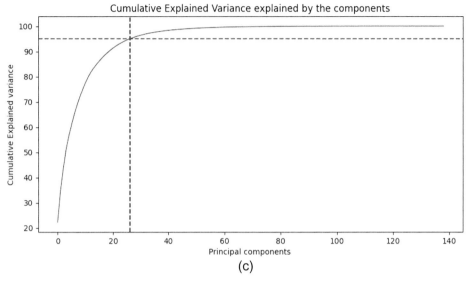

(c)

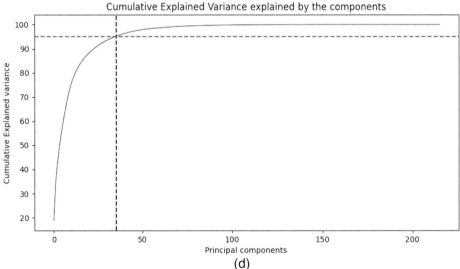

(d)

FIGURE 5.5 (Continued)

With an average of 70% compression, all the images can be viewed clearly. Until now, the IQA has been measured based on visual clarity, which is subjective. Hence, IQAs are measured tangibly by computing the MQS for all images, and can be seen in Table 5.2.

In Table 5.2, it can be noted that visibility attains with minimum component (*min_comp*) size of 39, 16, 26, and 35 out of 191-, 138-, 151-, and 234-pixel dimensions with the average original MQS (*MQS_or*) of 12.9. On a graded parametric study, it can be observed that with a *min_comp* size of 52, the clarity can be restored further with an average MQS post-compression (i.e., MQS_ac) of 10.8. With 70% average dimensionality reduction by PCA-based image compression and 16% gain in MQS on average, PCA can add a lot of value to lossless image compression.

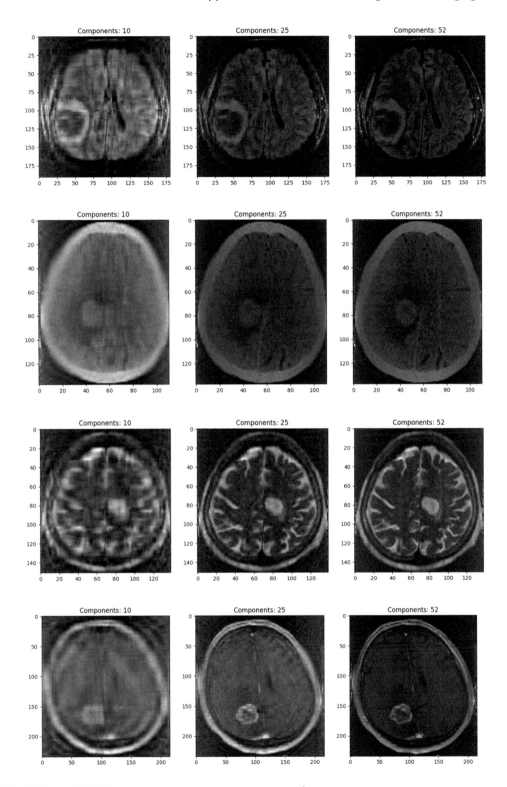

FIGURE 5.6   CT BRT image compression parametric study.

TABLE 5.2 A comprehensive view of CT BRT images concerning compression vs. MQS and the descriptive statistics (MQS_or = MQS of the original image and MQS_ac = MQS after compression)

Image	RGB_shape	GS_shape	Min_Comp	MQS_or	Min_comp (best clarity)	MQS_ac	Original_dim	Dim_reduction	MQS_gain
1	181 × 191 × 3	181 × 191	39	11.08	52	10.56	191	73%	5%
2	111 × 138 × 3	111 × 138	16	12.87		10	138	63%	22%
3	139 × 151 × 3	139 × 151	26	10.06		8.02	151	66%	20%
4	216 × 234 × 3	216 × 234	35	17.68		14.67	234	78%	16%
		Mean	29	12.9	52	10.8	178.5	70%	16%
		Median	30.5	11.9		10.2	171	70%	18%
		Stdev	10.2	3.37	0	2.79	43.33	7%	8%

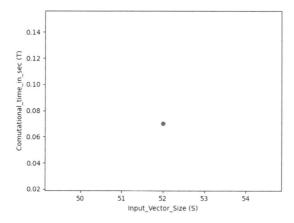

FIGURE 5.7 Big(O) plot.

5.4.6 Computational Time (Big(O))

Big(O) for CT BRT images with compressed pixel and original pixel size is plotted in Figure 5.7 for better clarity. It is important to note here that the numbers of compressed pixels are multiplied by 2 according to equation 5.4. Big(O) for male and female images is found to be linear with the size of pixels, which are crowded at around 52 components (represented by the hue).

The Big(O) plot shows a dot which is the common pointer to 52 components at which image clarity and quality can be preserved with the average timestamp of 0.07 s, which when compared to the average processing time of the original images is about 60% less time when compressed.

5.5 DISCUSSION

The chapter aims to handle the expected huge load of MRI and CT brain images with or without lesions as neuroimaging advances with time. An increasing number of image files each with a large size need to be reduced without much loss in the feature. It requires automatic analysis using PCA as an ML method as the human brain is unable to process multiple images simultaneously at any given timestamp. PCA is a mathematical technique that applies higher-order mathematical principles to convert the correlated variables into principal components, the smaller representation of the variables. In PCA the information contained (where high variances are detected) in a dataset is bagged with reduced dimensions. The integral projection of the dataset onto a subspace can be generated by a system of orthogonal axes. This reduces dimensions of the computational space and can represent data features significantly without much information loss. Such a reduction is a definitive advantage in image compression for automating the image processing method; principal components (as demarcated in the scree plots) can represent the data perfectly. PCA, hence, has been used for efficiently reducing the sizes of the images without losing important pixels, such as in CT BRT, as seen in this chapter. The size reduction is proportional to the time complexity of the computers, which the chapter has demonstrated successfully through a comprehensive step-by-step framework.

PCA has been used by several researchers for decades. A conventional comparative study of others' works with this work has been carefully avoided as the images used in those works are not the same as that used in this work. Hence, it cannot be correlated. Moreover, despite a rigorous search for studies where PCA has been used and the image compression percentage has been mentioned, it is not available to the best of the knowledge of the author. Having said that, in this section, an attempt has been made to examine some more studies where image compression is pursued from various medical and ML perspectives.

Apart from BRT feature processing, PCA has been successfully used in processing the brain images in various mental illnesses, such as schizophrenia, psychosis, mania, and attention deficit hyperactivity disorder, alongside the usage of principal components in various classification methods (supervised learning), e.g., regressions, SVM kernel, ANN, and so on, for screening and grading of diseases (Mwangi, Tian, & Soares, 2014). PCA also suffices for unsupervised learning as it does not need any class label assigned to the dependent variables that it studies (Mwangi, Tian, & Soares, 2014).

The drawbacks of PCA are (i) how many principal components one is looking for cannot be predefined and can cause a generalization error and to address that a cross-validation method is needed to find out the optimal number of principal components, (ii) as the principal components are the linear combination of the original features, its interpretation would be difficult, (iii) as the variance decreases eigenvalues are sorted in a descending manner, which may not reflect the practical importance of it, e.g., the differential aspect of disease to health or quality of life, (iv) as the principal components are derived from linear transformation, often they fail to represent and assess the nature of interaction and coupling among non-linear features, and finally (v) the disadvantage of ambiguous feature space creation while processing through voxels. In this aspect, it is important to mention that kernel PCA is a modified technique to create an optimum feature space using the kernel function (Mwangi, Tian, & Soares, 2014).

5.6 CONCLUSIONS AND FUTURE RESEARCH

This comprehensive study examines how efficiently PCA can be applied to compress CT BRT images ($N = 4$). Efficiency in image compression has been measured in two ways – (i) by visual impression of the reconstructed images, determined by 'clarity', which is subjective in nature and depends on one's visual acuity, and (ii) by MQS, which is an objective type of measure of the reconstructed images. It can be noted that with 70% average compression and average MQS of 10.8 (average MQS gain of 16%) reconstructed images can easily be visualized with the average component size of 52 against the average pixel size of 178.5. The gain in the processing speed on average is 60%. It is an encouraging result and can yield immediate insight on CT BRT images while automatic processing for the researchers, thereby saving time. The critical component size of 52 may further be evaluated with a larger image set. However, PCA can handle this additional information efficiently without any remarkable loss of data veracity.

It is suggested based on this study that PCA-based efficient compression (validated with MQS values) can be more appropriate in automated analyses of medical images for varieties of anomaly and pathology detection using ML and deep learning algorithms (Chattopadhyay, 2021, 2022). The *contribution* of the study lies on (i) systematic analysis of PCA on CT BRT images, (ii) its efficient compression, and disseminating the 'critical' size of the component to the researchers to save their time in finding the said value through tedious parametric study, (iii) a tangible way of measuring the compression efficiency using MQS, and (iv) disseminating the MQS gain among researchers. In automated image analysis in clinical care preservation of clinically significant image data is pivotal for accuracy in diagnosis, which can be achieved with less number of components much more efficiently using this methodology. It facilitates faster image processing retaining the important features intact.

The author recommends a larger study with many such images to note the critical component size of the CT BRT images.

REFERENCES

Abbas, A. H., Arab, A., & Harbi, J. (2018). Image Compression Using Principal Component Analysis. *Al-Mustansiriyah Journal of Science, 29*(2), 141–147.

Ai, D., Yang, J., Fan, J., Cong, W., & Wang, Y. (2015). Adaptive Tensor-Based Principal Component Analysis for Low-Dose CT Image Denoising. *PLOS ONE, 10*(5), e0126914.

American Cancer Society. (2020, May 5). Retrieved from What Causes Brain and Spinal Cord Tumors in Adults?: https://www.cancer.org/cancer/brain-spinal-cord-tumors-adults/causes-risks-prevention/what-causes.html

Azzarelli, R., Simons, B. D., & Philpott, A. (2018). The Developmental Origin of Brain Tumours: A Cellular and Molecular Framework. *Development, 145*(10), dev162693. https://doi.org/10.1242/dev.162693

Bhandary, A., Ananth Prabhu, G., Rajinikanth, V., Palani Thanaraj, K., Satapathy, S. C., Robbins, D. E., … Sri Madhava Raja, N. (2020). Deep-Learning Framework to Detect Lung Abnormality – A Study with Chest X-ray and Lung CT Scan Images. *Pattern Recognition Letters, 129*, 271–278.

Chattopadhyay, S. (2021). A Novel Approach to Detect Abnormal Chest X-rays of COVID-19 Patients Using Image Processing and Deep Learning. *Artificial Intelligence Evolution, 2*(2), 23–41. https://doi.org/10.37256/aie.222021977

Chattopadhyay, S. (2022). An Approach to Identify the Regions of Interest in Chest X-Ray Images of COVID-19 Patients and Its Clinical Validation. *Artificial Intelligence Evoluation, 3*(1), 41–54. https://doi.org/10.37256/aie.3120221331

Cleveland Clinic. (2022, February 6). Retrieved from Brain Cancer (Brain Tumor): https://my.clevelandclinic.org/health/diseases/6149-brain-cancer-brain-tumor#:~:text=Only%20about%20one%2Dthird%20of,brain%20are%20called%20primary%20tumors.

Diamantaras, K. I., & Kung, S. Y. (1996). *Principal Component Neural Networks: Theory and Applications.* John Wiley & Sons.

Doorsamy, W., & Rameshar, V. (2021). Investigation of PCA as a Compression Pre-Processing Tool for X-ray Image Classification. *Neural Computing and Applications.*

Hernandez, W., & Mendez, A. (2018, March 16). Application of Principal Component Analysis to Image Compression. In T. Göksel, *Statistics - Growing Data Sets and Growing Demand for Statistics.* IntechOpen. Retrieved April 17, 2021, from Application of Principal Component Analysis to Image Compression: Wilmar Hernandez and Alfredo Mendez (March 16th 2018). Application of Principal Component Analysis to Image Compression, Statistics - Growing Data Sets and Growing Demand for Statistics, Türkmen Göksel, IntechOpen, https://doi.org/10.5772/intechopen.75007.

Hotelling, H. (1933). Analysis of a Complex of Statistical Variables into Principal Components. *Journal of Educational Psychology, 24*(417–441), 498–520. https://doi.org/10.1037/h0071325

Jackson, J. E. (1991). *A User's Guide to Principal Components.* John Wiley & Sons. *John Hopkins Medicine.* (2022). Retrieved from Brain Tumors and Brain Cancer: https://www.hopkinsmedicine.org/health/conditions-and-diseases/brain-tumor

Jolliffe, I. T. (2002). *Principal Component Analysis.* 2nd ed. Springer.

Mao, T., Cuadros, A. P., Ma, X., He, W., Chen, Q., & Arce, G. R. (2019). Coded Aperture Optimization in X-Ray Tomography via Sparse Principal Component Analysis. *IEEE Transactions on Computational Imaging, 8*, 73–86.

Metwalli, M. R., Nasr, A. H., Farag Allah, O. S., & El-Rabaie, S. (2009). Image Fusion Based on Principal Component Analysis and High-Pass Filter. *2009 International Conference on Computer Engineering & Systems*, 63–70. Cairo, Egypt: IEEE.

Mohammed, S. B., Khalid, A., Osman, S. E., & Helali, R. G. (2016). Usage of Principal Component Analysis (PCA) in AI Applications. *International Journal of Engineering Research & Technology, 5*(12), 372–375.

Mwangi, B., Tian, T. S., & Soares, J. C. (2014). A Review of Feature Reduction Techniques in Neuroimaging. *Neuroinformatics, 12*(2), 229–244. https://doi.org/10.1007/s12021-013-9204-3

Nandi, D., Ashour, A. S., Samanta, S., Chakraborty, S., & Abdel-Megeed Mohammed Salem, M. (2015). Principal Component Analysis in Medical Image Processing: A Study. *International Journal of Image Mining, 1*(1), 45–64.

Narayan, P. (2019, May 8). *Why Private Scan Centres in Chennai Have Slashed Rates.* Retrieved from Times of India: https://timesofindia.indiatimes.com/city/chennai/why-private-scan-centres-in-chennai-have-slashed-rates/articleshow/69224821.cms

Ocampo, R. (2019, September 7). *Image Quality Assessment: A Survey.* Retrieved April 17, 2021, from https://ocampor.medium.com/advanced-methods-for-iqa-37581ec3c31f

Pearson, K. (1901). On Lines and Planes of Closest Fit to Systems of Points in Space. *Philosophical Magazine, 2*, 559–572. https://doi.org/10.1080/14786440109462720

Rasheed, J., Ali Hameed, A., Djeddi, C., Jamil, A., & Al-Turjman, F. (2021). A Machine Learning-Based Framework for Diagnosis of COVID-19 from Chest X-Ray Images. *Interdisciplinary Sciences: Computational Life Sciences, 13*, 103–117.

Roopa, H., & Asha, T. (2018). Feature Extraction of Chest X-ray Images and Analysis Using PCA and kPCA. *International Journal of Electrical and Computer Engineering, 8*(5), 3392–3398.

Saradha Rani, S., Sasibhushana Rao, G., & Prabhakara Rao, B. (2019). CT Scan and X-Ray Medical Images Compression using WDR and PCA techniques: A Performance Analysis. *International Journal of Recent Technology and Engineering, 7*(6), 2048–2051.

Schellekens, J. (2019, April 1). *questions/55438638/how-to-find-computation-complexity-of-image-processing-algorithm*. Retrieved April 17, 2021, from https://stackoverflow.com/: https://stackoverflow.com/questions/55438638/how-to-find-computation-complexity-of-image-processing-algorithm#:~:text=As%20a%20rough%20measure%2C%20you,viewed%2Fedited%20by%20the%20algorithm.&text=Its%20complexity%20is%20O(n,pixels%20in%20the%20input%20im

Shrimali, K. R. (2018, June 20). *Image Quality Assessment : BRISQUE*. Retrieved April 17, 2021, from Learn OpenCV: https://learnopencv.com/image-quality-assessment-brisque/

Sinha, U., & Kangarloo, H. (2002). Principal Component Analysis for Content-based Image Retrieval. *RadioGraphics, 22*(5), 1271–1289. https://doi.org/10.1148/radiographics.22.5.g02se021271. PMID: 12235353.

Taur, J. S., & Tao, C. (1996). Medical Image Compression Using Principal Component Analysis. *Proceedings of 3rd IEEE International Conference on Image Processing, 2*, 903–906. Lausanne, Switzerland: IEEE.

The Hindu. (2021, November 7). Retrieved from Cancer Institute Observes Brain Tumour Awareness Week: https://www.thehindu.com/news/national/tamil-nadu/cancer-institute-observes-brain-tumour-awareness-week/article37362750.ece

Vij, K., & Singh, Y. (2011). Enhancement of Images Using Histogram Processing Techniques. *INternational Journal of Computer Technology and Application, 2*(2), 309–313.

Wang, S.-H., Zhan, T.-M., Chen, Y., Zhang, Y., Yang, M., Lu, H.-M., … Phillips, P. (2016). Multiple Sclerosis Detection Based on Biorthogonal Wavelet Transform, RBF Kernel Principal Component Analysis, and Logistic Regression. *IEEE Access, 4*, 7567–7576.

Wichern, D. W., & Johnson, R. A. (2014). *Applied Multivariate Statistical Analysis*. 6th ed. Pearson Education Limited.

Yang, F., Hamit, M., Yan, C. B., Yao, J., Katluk, A., Kong, X. M., & Zhang, S. X. (2017). Feature Extraction and Classification on Esophageal X-Ray Images of Xinjiang Kazak Nationality. *Journal of Healthcare Engineering, 2017*(4620732). https://doi.org/10.1155/2017/4620732

CHAPTER 6

Role of Artificial Intelligence in Neuroimaging for Cognitive Research

Meenakshi Malviya, Alwin Joseph, Chandra J, and Pooja V

6.1 INTRODUCTION

Cognitive deficiency can be described as a mental impairment that affects various developmental activities at an early stage. A significant clinical irregularity can characterise an individual's intellectual and observational skills. The fastest-growing cognitive conditions at present are Alzheimer's disease (AD), Parkinson's disease (PD), autism spectrum disorder (ASD), attention deficit hyperactivity disorder (ADHD), and traumatic brain injury (TBI) [1, 2]. Diagnosis of cognitive impairments is possible with screening, interview, or questionnaire-based tools, but the recent trend is neuroimaging techniques. Neuroimaging is the study of the nervous system to understand cognitive disorders.

Neuroimaging such as magnetic resonance imaging (MRI), functional MRI (fMRI), computed tomography (CT), and positron emission tomography (PET) have been used in various cognitive disorders for better understanding [3]. The images provide anatomical and functional information to better understand and advance modern medicine. Neuroimaging modalities need experts to understand and interpret the data generated. Artificial intelligence (AI) has significantly improved the speed and accuracy of classification. AI has a vast collection of machine learning (ML) and deep learning (DL) algorithms [4]. AI strategies are applied to neuroimages as it needs an intensive study of each bit of information to understand the disorder. AI techniques include ML algorithms like decision trees, random forest, support vector machine (SVM), principal component analysis (PCA), and DL algorithms, including convolution neural networks (CNNs), long short-term memory (LSTM), and generative adversarial networks (GANs), which have wide applications for cognitive research.

DOI: 10.1201/9781003264767-6

AI can revolutionise the neuroimaging field for cognitive research by enabling more accurate and efficient analysis of large-scale datasets. Neuroimaging techniques, such as fMRI and PET, have allowed researchers to study the brain in unprecedented detail, but the sheer volume of data generated by these techniques can be overwhelming. AI techniques like ML and DL can help automate neuroimaging data analysis by identifying patterns and relationships that human analysts might miss. For example, ML algorithms are trained to classify different brain states based on activity patterns in fMRI scans. In contrast, DL algorithms can identify subtle changes in brain structure over time.

AI can also help to overcome some of the limitations of traditional neuroimaging techniques. For example, fMRI scans are subject to noise and artefacts that can interfere with the accuracy of the results. AI algorithms help to filter out these artefacts and improve the data quality. Additionally, AI can help to identify regions of interest in the brain that might be missed by human analysts, leading to more targeted and accurate studies.

Neuroimaging techniques have revolutionised the field of cognitive research by enabling us to visualise and understand the structure and function of the brain. However, analysing the vast amounts of data generated by neuroimaging studies can be time-consuming and laborious [5]. AI has powerful tools and techniques for processing and analysing large-scale neuroimaging data. AI algorithms can help to identify patterns and biomarkers associated with cognitive disorders, improve early diagnosis, and develop personalised treatment plans. Additionally, AI-powered tools, such as computerised cognitive training programmes and assistive technologies, can improve the treatment and management of cognitive disorders.

AI can transform neuroimaging for cognitive research by enabling more accurate and efficient analysis of large-scale datasets [6]. As AI technologies evolve, they will likely play an increasingly important role in advancing our understanding of the human brain and cognition. The chapter explains some of the most effective AI strategies, including ML and DL techniques, that can be applied to cognitive disorders using neuroimaging.

6.2 COGNITIVE DISORDERS

Cognitive disorders refer to conditions that affect an individual's cognitive abilities, such as thinking, memory, perception, and problem-solving. Various factors, including genetic predisposition, brain injury, infections, metabolic disorders, and other medical conditions, can cause these disorders. Some significant cognitive diseases are listed in Table 6.1 [7, 8].

TABLE 6.1   Commonly studied and identified cognitive disorders

Commonly studied and identified cognitive disorders
Alzheimer's disease (AD)
Parkinson's disease (PD)
Huntington's disease (HD)
Schizophrenia
Traumatic brain injury (TBI)
Attention deficit hyperactivity disorder (ADHD)
Autism spectrum disorder (ASD)

TABLE 6.2   Commonly studied neuroimaging techniques

Commonly studied neuroimaging techniques
Magnetic resonance imaging
Computed tomography
Positron emission tomography
Single-photon emission computed tomography
Electroencephalography
Diffusion tensor imaging

- *AD* is a progressive and irreversible neurological disorder affecting memory, thinking, and behaviour. It is the most common cause of dementia in older adults, accounting for up to 70% of cases. The disease typically starts with mild memory loss and progresses to more severe cognitive impairments, including language, reasoning, and decision-making difficulty. As the disease progresses, individuals may experience personality changes, mood swings, and difficulty with activities of daily living. The exact cause of AD is not yet fully understood, but it is caused due to complex interactions of genetic, environmental, and lifestyle factors. The condition is characterised by accumulating two abnormal brain proteins, beta-amyloid and tau. These proteins form clumps, called plaques and tangles, which interfere with communication between brain cells and eventually cause cell death. Medications help temporary improvements in the symptoms and slow the progression of AD. In addition, lifestyle changes, such as exercise and a healthy diet, may help to reduce the risk of developing AD [9, 10]. Due to the complexity of AD and the challenges associated with its diagnosis and treatment, there is a growing interest in using AI to improve understanding of the disease and develop new tools and treatments. AI algorithms help to identify patterns and biomarkers associated with the disease, predict disease progression, and develop personalised treatment plans. Additionally, AI-powered technologies help improve the quality of life of people with AD.

- *PD* is a degenerative disorder of the central nervous system that primarily affects movement but can also affect cognitive function. PD is a progressive neurological disorder affecting activity and other cognitive functions. The disease is caused by the loss of dopamine-producing cells in the brain, which leads to the characteristic motor symptoms of tremors, rigidity, and bradykinesia (slowness of movement). PD can also cause non-motor symptoms such as depression, anxiety, and cognitive impairment. The cause of PD is due to the complex interaction of genetic, environmental, and lifestyle factors. Medications and other therapies can help manage symptoms and improve the quality of life for people with PD. AI algorithms can analyse large amounts of data from various sources, including imaging, genetics, and patient records, to identify patterns and biomarkers associated with the disease. This can help to improve early diagnosis, track disease progression, and develop personalised treatment plans. AI-powered technologies, such as wearables and smart home devices, can also be used to monitor and manage the symptoms of PD [11, 12]. For example, wearables can track tremors and other motor symptoms. At the same time, smart home devices can assist with activities of daily living and provide a safe and comfortable living environment for individuals with PD.

- *Huntington's disease (HD)* is a genetic disorder that causes progressive deterioration of the nerve cells in the brain, leading to involuntary movements, emotional problems, and cognitive impairment. HD is a rare, progressive neurological disorder that causes the degeneration of brain cells, particularly in the basal ganglia, resulting in various motor, cognitive, and psychiatric symptoms. The disease is inherited in an autosomal dominant pattern, meaning a person only needs to inherit one copy of the mutated gene from either parent to develop the disease. The symptoms of HD include chorea (involuntary movements), dystonia (muscle contractions), rigidity, and problems with coordination and balance. As HD progresses, cognitive and psychiatric symptoms such as memory loss, difficulty concentrating, depression, and irritability may also occur. HD treatments focus on managing symptoms and improving quality of life. AI has the potential to aid in the diagnosis, monitoring, and treatment of HD [13, 14]. AI algorithms can analyse large amounts of data, including brain imaging and genetic data, to identify patterns and biomarkers associated with the disease. It can improve early diagnosis and tracking of disease progression, which can help guide treatment decisions. AI-powered technologies assist individuals with HD in their daily activities, improving their quality of life. Wearable devices can track symptoms such as tremors and gait disturbances, providing valuable information to healthcare providers for individualised care plans. AI-powered drug discovery platforms can rapidly screen large databases of compounds to identify potential therapeutic targets, which can then be further tested and developed into new medications.

- *Schizophrenia* is a chronic and severe mental disorder that affects how a person thinks, feels, and behaves. People with schizophrenia often experience delusions, hallucinations, disordered thinking, and cognitive deficits. Schizophrenia is a severe and chronic mental disorder that affects approximately 1% of the population worldwide. Schizophrenia occurs due to a complex interplay between genetic, environmental, and developmental factors [15, 16]. AI has the potential to aid in the diagnosis, monitoring, and treatment of schizophrenia. AI algorithms can analyse large amounts of data from various sources, including imaging, genetics, and patient records, to identify patterns and biomarkers associated with the disease. This can help improve early diagnosis and personalised treatment plans for individuals with schizophrenia. AI-powered technologies help to simulate and treat the symptoms of schizophrenia. For example, virtual reality can simulate situations that trigger paranoia or anxiety, allowing individuals with schizophrenia to practise coping strategies in a safe and controlled environment. Chatbots can provide cognitive behavioural therapy and other forms of psychotherapy to individuals with schizophrenia, providing support and guidance outside traditional therapy settings. Moreover, AI helps to develop new treatments for schizophrenia. AI-powered drug discovery platforms can rapidly screen large databases of compounds to identify potential therapeutic targets, which can then be further tested and developed into new medications for persons with schizophrenia.

- *TBI* is a brain injury caused by a blow or jolt to the head, which can cause cognitive impairments such as memory loss, attention problems, and difficulty with problem-solving. TBIs can range from mild, with symptoms such as headache and temporary confusion, to severe, with symptoms such as seizures, coma, and death. TBI can have long-lasting effects on cognitive, emotional, and physical functioning. AI has the potential to aid in the diagnosis, monitoring, and treatment of TBI [17, 18]. AI algorithms can analyse large amounts of data, including brain imaging and patient records, to identify patterns and biomarkers associated with the severity and progression of TBI. This can help improve early diagnosis and personalised treatment plans for individuals with TBI. AI-powered technologies enable to monitor and manage the symptoms of TBI. For example, wearable devices can track physical activity and sleep patterns, providing valuable information to healthcare providers for individualised care plans. Mobile apps can also provide cognitive and behavioural therapy to individuals with TBI, helping to improve memory and other cognitive functions. AI helps to develop new treatments for TBI. AI-powered drug discovery platforms can rapidly screen large databases of compounds to identify potential therapeutic targets, which can then be further tested and developed into new medications.

- *ADHD* is a neurodevelopmental disorder characterised by inattention, hyperactivity, and impulsivity. It can affect cognitive function, particularly in attention and working memory. ADHD can significantly impact academic, social, and occupational functioning, leading to comorbid conditions such as anxiety and depression. AI has the potential to aid in the diagnosis, monitoring, and treatment of ADHD [19, 20]. AI algorithms can analyse large amounts of data from various sources, including brain imaging, behavioural assessments, and genetics, to identify patterns and biomarkers associated with the disorder. This can help improve early diagnosis and personalised treatment plans for individuals with ADHD. AI-powered technologies allow us to simulate and treat the symptoms of ADHD. For example, virtual reality can be used to improve attention and focus through cognitive training exercises. Mobile apps can provide cognitive behavioural therapy and other forms of psychotherapy to individuals with ADHD, providing support and guidance outside of traditional therapy settings. AI can be used to develop new treatments for ADHD. AI-powered drug discovery platforms can rapidly screen large databases of compounds to identify potential therapeutic targets, which can then be further tested and developed into new medications.

- *ASD* is a developmental disorder that affects social communication, interaction, behaviour, and interests. Individuals with ASD often have cognitive impairments in social cognition and executive function. ASD is a complex disorder with many symptoms and severity, challenging diagnosis and treatment. AI has the potential to aid in the diagnosis and treatment of ASD [21, 22]. AI algorithms can analyse large amounts of data from various sources, including brain imaging, behavioural assessments, and genetics, to identify patterns and biomarkers associated with the disorder. This can help improve early diagnosis and personalised treatment plans for individuals with ASD. AI-powered technologies, such as wearable devices and mobile apps, can also be used to monitor and manage the symptoms of ASD. For example, wearable devices can track physiological signals, such as heart rate and skin conductance, providing valuable information to healthcare providers for individualised care plans. Mobile apps can provide cognitive and behavioural therapy to individuals with ASD, helping to improve social skills and other areas of functioning. Moreover, AI can be used to develop new treatments for ASD. AI-powered drug discovery platforms can rapidly screen large databases of compounds to identify potential therapeutic targets, which can then be further tested and developed into new medications.

Treatment for cognitive disorders can vary depending on the underlying cause and severity of the symptoms. AI is applied to identify and generate tools for supporting people with these disorders [23, 24]. Applications of AI solutions include medications, behavioural therapy, cognitive rehabilitation, and lifestyle change support. Early diagnosis and intervention can help to manage symptoms and improve outcomes for individuals with cognitive disorders. AI tools help quickly identify these neurological disorders and help the patients with solutions for their support and treatment.

6.3 NEUROIMAGING TECHNIQUES

Neuroimaging can be structural/functional imaging. Structural images provide the detailed structure of the brain. MRI, CT, and SPECT (single-photon emission computed tomography) generate structural images of the brain. Functional imaging captures brain images during some activity, for example, fMRI and EEG (electroencephalography) [3, 25]. MRI is beneficial in detecting structural changes in the brain associated with cognitive disorders. PET and SPECT can detect changes in brain metabolism and blood flow. SPECT scan is used to detect altered blood flow in the brain. A SPECT scan is a nuclear medicine exam that uses a radioactive compound to diagnose some brain diseases. Generally, neuroimaging is a non-invasive process, but PET and SPECT are invasive tests due to a dose of radioactive material before the test.

However, interpreting these imaging data requires a high level of expertise. Various studies and their findings prove that neuroimaging has a promising future in research and psychiatric diagnosis. The significance of neuroimaging in cognitive studies has increased exponentially for multiple applications, including diagnosis, localisation of cognitive function, monitoring treatment and research, etc. Some neuroimaging techniques commonly used to diagnose cognitive deficiencies are listed in Table 6.1, and a detailed summary of neuroimaging techniques applied in various cognitive studies is concluded in Figure 6.1.

- *MRI* is a non-invasive imaging technique that uses strong magnetic fields and radio waves to generate detailed images of the body's internal structures. MRI is a widely used neuroimaging technique to study the structure and function of the brain in

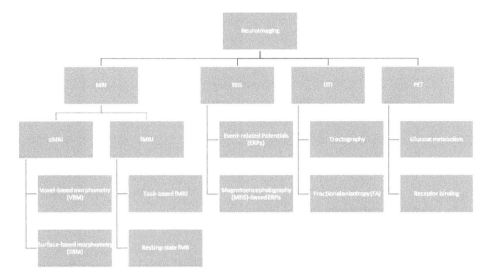

FIGURE 6.1   Summary of neuroimaging applied in cognitive neuroscience.

health and disease. MRI has revolutionised the field of cognitive neuroscience, helping to study the brain in vivo without the need for invasive procedures [26]. MRI helps to study brain structure, function, and connectivity, allowing for a better understanding of how the brain supports cognitive processes such as perception, attention, memory, and decision-making. Functional MRI (fMRI) is a specific type of MRI that measures changes in blood oxygenation levels in the brain, which are associated with neural activity. fMRI can identify active brain regions during specific cognitive tasks, providing insights into the neural basis of cognition. Diffusion MRI (dMRI) is another type used to study the connectivity of the brain's white matter. dMRI measures the diffusion of water molecules in the brain's white matter, which provides information about the orientation and integrity of neural fibres. dMRI helps to study the connections between different brain regions, providing insights into the neural networks that underlie cognitive processes. MRI has also been used in cognitive research to study the effects of various diseases and conditions on the brain, including AD, PD, TBI, and psychiatric disorders such as schizophrenia and depression [27].

- *CT* is a non-invasive imaging technique that uses X-rays to produce detailed images of the body's internal structures. CT is used in neuroimaging to study the brain's structure in health and disease. CT provides detailed images of the brain's structure, shape, size, and density. CT is beneficial for identifying brain lesions and other abnormalities, such as tumours or areas of haemorrhage, that can affect cognitive function. CT can also study the effects of different diseases and conditions on the brain, such as TBI, stroke, and neurodegenerative disorders like AD and PD. CT cannot directly visualise the brain's functional activity or neural connections. CT exposes patients to ionising radiation, which can be harmful at high doses. As a result, CT is generally used less frequently than MRI in cognitive research [28]. CT remains a valuable tool in neuroimaging for cognitive research, particularly the structural abnormalities in the brain to be assessed and in emergencies where rapid diagnosis is essential.

- *PET* is a non-invasive imaging technique that uses radioactive tracers to study the metabolic and biochemical processes of the body, including the brain. PET helps to study brain function and activity in health and disease. PET measures the distribution and uptake of radioactive tracers, usually injected into the bloodstream. The tracers bind to specific molecules in the brain, such as glucose or neurotransmitters, associated with brain activity. PET can study changes in brain activity in response to cognitive tasks and changes in brain metabolism and neurotransmitter function in different disease states. PET can study various cognitive processes, including perception, attention, memory, language, and emotion. It has been used extensively in the study of neurodegenerative disorders, such as AD, PD, and HD, to understand these conditions' underlying pathophysiology better. PET can also study psychiatric disorders such as depression, anxiety, and schizophrenia. PET has several advantages over other neuroimaging techniques, including its ability to measure changes in brain activity in real time and its high sensitivity to changes in brain metabolism and neurotransmitter function [29]. PET is limited by its relatively low spatial resolution and the need for exposure to ionising radiation, which can be harmful at high doses.

- *SPECT* is a nuclear medicine imaging technique used to study blood flow and metabolism. SPECT is used in neuroimaging to study brain function and activity in health and disease. SPECT measures the distribution and uptake of a radioactive tracer injected into the bloodstream. The tracer emits gamma rays, which are detected by a gamma camera that rotates around the head to create a 3D image of the brain. SPECT allows studying changes in brain activity and blood flow in response to cognitive tasks and changes in brain metabolism and blood flow in different disease states. SPECT can study various cognitive processes, including perception, attention, memory, language, and emotion. It has been used extensively in the study of neurodegenerative disorders, such as AD, PD, and HD, to understand these conditions' underlying pathophysiology better [30]. SPECT can also study psychiatric disorders such as depression, anxiety, and schizophrenia. SPECT has several advantages over other neuroimaging techniques, including its ability to measure changes in brain activity and blood flow in real time, its relative affordability, and its widespread availability. SPECT is limited by its relatively low spatial resolution, which can limit its ability to localise brain activity accurately, and by the need for exposure to ionising radiation.

- *EEG* is a non-invasive neuroimaging technique that measures the brain's electrical activity using electrodes placed on the scalp. EEG is used to study brain function and activity in health and disease. EEG measures the electrical signals generated by neurons in the brain and provides a real-time measure of brain activity. EEG studies changes in brain activity in response to cognitive tasks and changes in brain activity in different disease states. EEG helps to study various cognitive processes, including perception, attention, memory, language, and emotion. EEG is extensively used to study neurodegenerative disorders like AD, PD, and HD to better understand these conditions' underlying pathophysiology. EEG can also study psychiatric disorders such as depression, anxiety, and schizophrenia [31]. EEG has several advantages over other neuroimaging techniques, including its high temporal resolution, which allows for measuring changes in brain activity in real time, and its relatively low cost and portability. EEG is limited by its relatively low spatial resolution, limiting its ability to localise brain activity accurately.

- *Diffusion tensor imaging (DTI)* is a type of MRI used to study the structure and connectivity of white matter in the brain. In cognitive research, DTI is used to study the connections between different brain regions and their role in cognitive processes. DTI measures the movement and diffusion of water molecules in white matter tracts in the brain. DTI creates images of the white matter tracts and measures their integrity and connectivity by measuring the direction and speed of water diffusion. DTI helps to study various cognitive processes, including perception, attention, memory, language, and emotion. It has been used extensively in the study of neurodegenerative disorders, such as AD, PD, and HD, to understand these conditions' underlying pathophysiology better. DTI can also be used to study psychiatric disorders such as depression, anxiety, and schizophrenia [32]. DTI has several advantages over other neuroimaging techniques, including its ability to visualise the structural connections between different brain regions and its sensitivity to changes in white matter integrity. Its relatively low spatial resolution limits DTI and its inability to provide information about the functional activity of the brain.

6.4 AI FOR COGNITIVE DISORDERS

AI in medicine started in 1950, about five decades ago. The seminal transformation. The advancement of technology evolved AI in medicine in various fields. Neuroimaging is the most recent development to aid in the early and accurate identification of cognitive disorders. ML and DL algorithms have been used to analyse MRI, PET, and SPECT data to identify patterns associated with cognitive disorders. AI is applicable in various fields of cognitive study using medical imaging:

- ML algorithms: ML algorithms are being used to develop predictive models for cognitive disorders such as AD. These algorithms analyse extensive brain imaging, genetic, and clinical data datasets to identify patterns and biomarkers associated with cognitive impairment. These models can help to predict the onset and progression of cognitive disorders, identify at-risk individuals, and improve early diagnosis. ML algorithms like decision trees, random forests, SVM, and PCA have numerous applications in cognitive research. DL algorithms, including CNN, LSTM, and GANs, also help in cognitive research [33].

- Natural language processing (NLP) algorithms: NLP algorithms are used to analyse language patterns in individuals with cognitive disorders such as schizophrenia and autism. These algorithms can help identify linguistic markers associated with cognitive impairment and provide insights into the cognitive processes underlying these disorders. NLP helps in the effortless analysis of text-based data gathered for cognitive disorders. NLP can be applied to perform text classification, sentiment analysis, language modelling, and information extraction [34].

- Computerised cognitive training: AI algorithms are used to develop automated cognitive training programmes for individuals with cognitive impairments. These programmes use ML algorithms to adapt to an individual's cognitive abilities and provide targeted training to improve cognitive function. Cognitive disorders relating to attention, memory, and executive function use computerised cognitive training as a mechanism of treatment and care [35].

- Virtual assistants: AI-powered virtual assistants, such as chatbots, are used to support and assist individuals with cognitive disorders. These assistants can provide reminders, answer questions, and offer emotional support, improving the quality of life for individuals with cognitive impairments [35].

- Robotics: AI-powered robots are being developed to assist individuals with cognitive disorders in daily meal preparation, medication management, and mobility. These robots use ML algorithms to adapt to an individual's needs and preferences and provide personalised assistance.

- Image analysis: AI algorithms analyse medical images such as X-rays, CT scans, and MRIs to identify abnormalities or patterns indicative of a specific disease. ML algorithms are trained on large datasets of medical images to recognise complex patterns complicated for radiologists to detect manually.

- Automated diagnosis: AI algorithms help to identify abnormalities or patterns in medical images to diagnose diseases automatically. This can significantly improve the efficiency of disease classification and reduce the need for human intervention.

- Patient triage: AI algorithms triage patients based on severity levels for faster treatment planning.

- Treatment planning: AI algorithms are helpful for clinicians in developing treatment plans for patients with specific diseases. The algorithms are prepared to analyse the patient's medical images to identify the severity and suitable course of treatment.

- Prediction: The significance of AI algorithms is more in the projection and identification of the progression of diseases based on medical images with more accurate prognoses.

AI algorithms and techniques offer great potential for developing new tools and technologies to improve cognitive disorders' diagnosis, treatment, and management. As AI technologies continue to advance, we will see an increasing number of innovative applications for these algorithms in the field of cognitive disorders [36, 37]. The various cognitive disorders require individualised treatment plans and medication. Patient care can be optimised with the help of AI tools to predict and forecast the patient's reaction towards medication and treatments.

6.4.1 ML for Neuroimaging

We present a review on ML methods to predict conversion from mild cognitive impairment (MCI) to AD. The authors discuss various techniques used to predict disease progression, such as SVMs and random forests, as well as different types of imaging data used for analysis, such as structural MRI and Fluorodeoxyglucose (FDG)-positron emission tomography (PET). The authors conclude that ML methods have shown promise for predicting disease progression in MCI. Future studies should focus on standardising imaging protocols and exploring the use of multimodal data for improved prediction accuracy [38].

Multimodal feature selection and fusion approach for AD diagnosis using MRI and FDG-PET imaging data is presented. The authors use a genetic algorithm to select the most relevant features from each modality and then combine them using a SVM classifier. The authors evaluate their approach on a dataset of 120 individuals with AD and 120 age-matched healthy controls, achieving high classification accuracy, sensitivity, and specificity. The authors also demonstrate that the selected features are biologically meaningful and relevant to AD pathology. Overall, the study highlights the potential of combining multiple imaging modalities for improved diagnosis of AD and the importance of feature selection for reducing the dimensionality of the data and improving classification accuracy [39].

ML is all about training computers according to human needs. The trained computer recognises a pattern in the data and also learns from experience. The process of jif teaching computers is based on two methods termed as labelled supervised learning and unlabelled unsupervised learning. Supervised learning is the categorised data that is being used for training. Unsupervised data is considered the raw data, and it looks for patterns and pattern matches to the data. Reinforcement learning learns from its mistakes. ML has many applications, including NLP, image recognition, recommendation systems, fraud detection, and autonomous vehicles. Many techniques are increasingly popular in analysing neuroimaging data due to their ability to detect subtle patterns in complex data [40].

- **SVM**: An SVM is a supervised learning algorithm for classification and regression tasks. They are mainly used in neuroimage research because they can handle high-dimensional data and find complex patterns in brain imaging data.

  They identify the hyperplane that best separates the different classes in the data [41].

  Maximise 1/2 ||w||^2 subject to y_i(w.T xi + b) >= 1 for all I

  where w is the weight vector, b is the bias term, x_i is the input vector, and y_i is the output label (+1 or −1).

  SVM has been used to classify brain images into cognitive disorders such as AD, PD, and schizophrenia. SVM can also identify brain regions most important for distinguishing between cognitive disorders. The advantage of SVM in neuroimaging is its ability to handle high-dimensional data with many features. SVM can also identify subtle patterns and features in brain images that are not easily discernible by visual inspection.

- **Independent component analysis (ICA):** ICA is not an unsupervised learning algorithm; it is used to identify sources contributing to a set of observations. ICA is beneficial in neuroimaging research because it can separate brain signals from noise and artefacts in fMRI data.

  X = AS

  where X is the observed data, A is the mixing matrix, and S is the set of independent sources.

  ICA decomposes fMRI data into independent components, spatially and temporally distinct patterns of brain activity. Each independent component represents a unique source of neural activity in the brain, and ICA can identify multiple independent components that are active simultaneously. ICA has several advantages in neuroimaging research. It is a data-driven approach that requires no prior assumptions about the underlying activity sources. This makes ICA useful for exploring new hypotheses and identifying novel patterns of brain activity. ICA can identify spatially and temporally distinct patterns of activity that may not be visible using traditional methods of fMRI analysis. ICA can separate task-related from task-unrelated neural activity, which is important for identifying brain regions involved in a particular cognitive task.

- **Random forest:** Random forest is a learning method for classification and regression tasks. It works by combining multiple decision trees to improve the accuracy and robustness of the final model. Random forest algorithm can handle high-dimensional data with many features, such as brain images. Random forest has been used to classify brain images into different cognitive disorders, such as AD and PD. Random forest can also identify brain regions most important for distinguishing between cognitive disorders.

- **PCA: PCA** is an unsupervised learning technique used to reduce the dimensionality of neuroimaging data; it identifies the main component of the data, which can be used to input future data for another ML algorithm [41]. PCA is often used to reduce the number of variables and identify the most important features or patterns of brain activity associated with cognitive function or cognitive disorders. PCA can also explore the relationships between different brain regions and cognitive tasks. The advantage of PCA in neuroimaging is its ability to reduce the noise and variability in the data, making it easier to identify the most relevant features or patterns of brain activity. PCA can also help identify brain regions most important for specific cognitive tasks or disorders.

Apart from the algorithms mentioned above, many ML algorithms facilitate the study, detection, and classification of cognitive and neurological disorders. ML algorithms like decision trees, random forests, SVMs, and PCA help in the processing of data gathered from various sources that help in the prognosis of cognitive disorders.

6.4.2 DL for Neuroimaging

A DL model uses raw imaging data to predict brain age. The discriminating features were reported as a reliable and heritable biomarker associated with cognitive performance, brain structure, and genetic variants. The study demonstrates the potential of DL methods for predicting biomarkers of brain ageing from raw imaging data [42]. Neuroimaging and AI techniques have shown great promise in identifying cognitive diseases such as AD, PD, and other forms of dementia. In this literature review, we will discuss recent studies that have explored the use of neuroimaging and AI in identifying cognitive diseases.

- **Convolutional neural network (CNN)**: CNN is a DL algorithm useful for image analysis tasks. CNN uses a hierarchical architecture to automatically extract relevant features from the images and be used for tasks such as image segmentation and object recognition [43].

  f_i = activation function ($\sum w_{ij} * x_{i+j-1} + b_i$)

  where f_i is the output feature map, w_{ij} is the weight matrix for the jth filter, x_{i+j-1} is the input to the jth filter, and b_i is the bias term.

  The study demonstrates the potential of combining multiple imaging modalities and advanced feature learning methods for improved multiclass diagnosis of neuro-degenerative diseases like ASD, PD, and other cognitive deficiencies.

- **Deep belief networks** (DBNs): This type of DL algorithm is an unsupervised learning task; it composes the multiple layers of restricted bold transmission DBN and uses it to extract features from the neuroimage in data. Various techniques are used in the neuroimaging task, including brain image segmentation, classification of brain regions, and prediction of clinical outcomes.

  DL algorithms gain knowledge by processing data at progressively higher levels of abstraction, emphasising DL for image classification and image segmentation in neuroimaging. A deep understanding of computer vision has had the most success out of all the ML applications in medicine [44]. CNN can help in image segmentation and classification of neuroimages. DL and ML are increasingly used in the clinical workflow and the interpretation of neuroimaging [45].

- **Recurrent neural networks (RNNs)**: RNNs are a DL algorithm that models data sequences, such as time-series data. RNNs have been used to analyse functional magnetic resonance imaging (fMRI) data and to predict disease progression in AD.

- **GANs**: GANs are a type of DL algorithm designed to generate new data samples similar to the training data. GANs have been used to generate synthetic brain images to train and validate other DL algorithms.

- **Autoencoders**: Autoencoders are a DL algorithm designed to learn a compressed data representation. Autoencoders have been used for tasks such as denoising fMRI data and identifying abnormal brain regions in AD.

Apart from the algorithms mentioned above, many DL algorithms facilitate the study, detection, and classification of cognitive and neurological disorders. DL algorithms, including CNNs, LSTM, and GANs, help in the processing of the data that has been gathered from various sources for studying cognitive and neurological disorders.

6.5 ROLE OF DL AND ML IN COGNITIVE DISORDERS

DL and ML are two powerful branches of AI increasingly used to develop new tools and technologies for cognitive disorders. Here are some examples of the role of DL and ML in cognitive disorders:

- *Diagnosis*: DL and ML algorithms can analyse extensive brain imaging, genetic, and clinical data datasets to identify patterns and biomarkers associated with cognitive disorders. These algorithms can be used to develop predictive models to identify individuals at risk of developing cognitive disorders and improve early diagnosis.

- *Treatment*: DL and ML algorithms can be used to develop personalised treatment plans for individuals with cognitive disorders. These algorithms can analyse various factors, such as an individual's medical history, genetic makeup, and lifestyle, to develop treatment plans tailored to their needs and preferences.

- *Monitoring*: DL and ML algorithms can be used to monitor the progression of cognitive disorders and track the effectiveness of treatments. These algorithms can analyse changes in brain imaging, behavioural data, and other biomarkers to provide insights into disease progression and treatment response.

- *Computerised cognitive training*: DL and ML algorithms can be used to develop computerised cognitive training programmes for individuals with cognitive impairments. These programmes use ML algorithms to adapt to an individual's cognitive abilities and provide targeted training to improve cognitive function.

- *Assistive technologies*: DL and ML algorithms can be used to develop assistive technologies for individuals with cognitive impairments. These technologies can include virtual assistants, robots, and other devices that use ML algorithms to provide personalised support and assistance.

DL and ML algorithms offer great potential for developing new tools and technologies to improve diagnosis, treatment, and management. As these technologies evolve, we will likely see more innovative applications for DL and ML in cognitive disorders.

6.6 CHALLENGES AND FUTURE DIRECTION

Developing ML/DL predictive models for various brain disorders requires an appropriate selection of pre-processing techniques, feature extraction and selection methods, and classification strategies. Numerous predictive models have been developed. However, real-time implementation for professionals is not yet achieved due to challenges such as heterogeneity within diagnostic categories and variability in imaging protocols and data quality. The promises and potential pitfalls of single-subject prediction of brain disorders in neuroimaging are discussed in detail [46].

Neuroimaging is a valuable tool for studying the structure and function of the brain. It is a recent trend in healthcare for various significant contributions such as diagnosis of deficiencies, understanding the neuropathology, treatment planning, and investigating other effects of the present condition. Some technical challenges with neuroimaging require complex and expensive equipment and specialised training to operate and analyse the resulting data. Some more concerns to be monitored are ethical considerations, participant recruitment, data analysis, interpretation of findings, and replication and generalizability.

The authors also highlight the challenges and limitations of neuroimaging-based classification studies, such as sample size and variability, cross-validation, and generalizability. The review provides a comprehensive overview of the current neuroimaging-based classification studies for AD and its prodromal stages. It also identifies future research directions for improving accuracy and clinical relevance [47].

While the role of AI in neuroimaging for cognitive research holds great potential, several challenges need to be addressed. Here are some of the critical challenges and future directions for this field:

- *Data quality and quantity*: One of the significant challenges in using AI algorithms for cognitive research is the availability of high-quality and large-scale datasets. Efforts are needed to collect more standardised and well-annotated datasets that can be used to train and validate AI algorithms.

- *Interoperability*: The need for interoperability between different neuroimaging platforms and tools can hinder the development of AI algorithms that can be used across different research settings. Efforts are needed to standardise neuroimaging protocols and promote data sharing across research teams.

- *Generalisation*: Many AI algorithms are developed and validated on a single dataset or a single task, which can limit their generalizability to new settings and functions. Efforts are needed to create more robust and generalisable AI algorithms that can be applied to different cognitive research questions and datasets.

- *Ethical considerations*: Using AI algorithms in cognitive research raises significant ethical concerns, such as privacy, informed consent, and bias. Future research should address these ethical issues and develop guidelines for the responsible use of AI in cognitive research.

In the future, the field of AI in neuroimaging for cognitive research is expected to grow rapidly. New AI algorithms and tools will be developed to improve the accuracy and efficiency of cognitive assessments and to assist in developing new treatments for cognitive disorders. As AI technologies evolve, addressing the challenges and ethical considerations associated with their use is essential to ensure that the potential benefits are realised while minimising any negative impact on individuals and society.

6.7 CONCLUSION

The study provides empirical evidence for the utility of structural brain MRI scans to predict cognitive deficiencies and their prodromal stages. The role of AI in neuroimaging for cognitive research is rapidly expanding. AI algorithms are being used to analyse extensive brain imaging, genetic, and clinical data datasets to identify patterns and biomarkers associated with cognitive disorders. These algorithms can help predict the onset and progression of cognitive disorders, identify at-risk individuals, and improve early diagnosis.

ML algorithms include decision trees, random forest, SVM, PCA, and DL algorithms, such as CNNs, LSTM, and GANs. Additionally, AI-powered tools and technologies, such as computerised cognitive training programmes and assistive technologies, are being developed to improve the treatment and management of cognitive disorders. As AI technologies advance, we will likely see an increasing number of innovative applications for these algorithms in cognitive disorders, ultimately leading to improved outcomes for individuals with cognitive impairments.

REFERENCES

[1] Giri, Mohan, et al. "Prevalence and correlates of cognitive impairment and depression among elderly people in the world's fastest growing city, Chongqing, People's Republic of China." *Clinical Interventions in Aging* (2016): 1091–1098. doi: 10.2147/CIA.S113668. PMID: 27574409; PMCID: PMC4990376

[2] Haan, Mary N., and Minda Weldon. "The influence of diabetes, hypertension, and stroke on ethnic differences in physical and cognitive functioning in an ethnically diverse older population." *Annals of Epidemiology* 6.5 (1996): 392–398.

[3] Aine, Cheryl J. "A conceptual overview and critique of functional neuroimaging techniques in humans: I. MRI/FMRI and PET." *Critical Reviews in Neurobiology* 9.2–3 (1995): 229–309.

[4] Serra, Angela, Paola Galdi, and Roberto Tagliaferri. "Machine learning for bioinformatics and neuroimaging." *Wiley Interdisciplinary Reviews: Data Mining and Knowledge Discovery* 8.5 (2018): e1248.

[5] Mayberg, Helen S. "Neuroimaging and psychiatry: the long road from bench to bedside." *Hastings Center Report* 44.s2 (2014): S31–S36.

[6] Allen, Bryce L. "Cognitive research in information science: implications for design." *Annual Review of Information Science and Technology* 26 (1991): 3–37.

[7] Monk, Terri G., and Catherine C. Price. "Postoperative cognitive disorders." *Current Opinion in Critical Care* 17.4 (2011): 376–381. doi: 10.1097/MCC.0b013e328348bece.

[8] McWhirter, Laura, Craig Ritchie, Jon Stone, and Alan Carson. "Functional cognitive disorders: a systematic review." *The Lancet Psychiatry* 7.2 (2020, Feb. 1): 191–207.

[9] Scheltens, Philip, Kaj Blennow, Monique MB Breteler, Bart De Strooper, Giovanni B. Frisoni, Stephen Salloway, and Wiesje Maria Van der Flier. "Alzheimer's disease." *The Lancet* 388.10043 (2016): 505–517.

[10] Ballard, Clive, Serge Gauthier, Anne Corbett, Carol Brayne, Dag Aarsland, and Emma Jones. "Alzheimer's disease." *The Lancet* 377.9770 (2011): 1019–1031.

[11] Bloem, Bastiaan R., Michael S. Okun, and Christine Klein. "Parkinson's disease." *The Lancet* 397.10291 (2021): 2284–2303.

[12] Lang, Anthony E., and Andres M. Lozano. "Parkinson's disease." *New England Journal of Medicine* 339.16 (1998): 1130–1143.

[13] Walker, Francis O. "Huntington's disease." *The Lancet* 369.9557 (2007): 218–228.

[14] Ha, Ainhi D., and Victor S.C. Fung. "Huntington's disease." *Current Opinion in Neurology* 25.4 (2012): 491–498.

[15] McCutcheon, Robert A., Tiago Reis Marques, and Oliver D. Howes. "Schizophrenia—an overview." *JAMA Psychiatry* 77.2 (2020): 201–210.

[16] Osmond, Humphry, and John Smythies. "Schizophrenia: a new approach." *Journal of Mental Science* 98.411 (1952): 309–315.

[17] Ghajar, Jamshid. "Traumatic brain injury." *The Lancet* 356.9233 (2000): 923–929.

[18] Finnie, J. W., and P. C. Blumbergs. "Traumatic brain injury." *Veterinary Pathology* 39.6 (2002): 679–689.

[19] Wender, Paul H. "Attention-deficit hyperactivity disorder in adults." *Psychiatric Clinics of North America* 21.4 (1998): 761–774.

[20] Faraone, Stephen V., Joseph Biederman, Thomas Spencer, Tim Wilens, Larry J. Seidman, Eric Mick, and Alysa E. Doyle. "Attention-deficit/hyperactivity disorder in adults: an overview." *Biological Psychiatry* 48.1 (2000): 9–20.

[21] Lord, Catherine, Mayada Elsabbagh, Gillian Baird, and Jeremy Veenstra-Vanderweele. "Autism spectrum disorder." *The Lancet* 392.10146 (2018): 508–520.

[22] Faras, Hadeel, Nahed Al Ateeqi, and Lee Tidmarsh. "Autism spectrum disorders." *Annals of Saudi Medicine* 30.4 (2010): 295–300.

[23] Battineni, Gopi, et al. "Artificial intelligence models in the diagnosis of adult-onset dementia disorders: a review." *Bioengineering* 9.8 (2022): 370.

[24] Mirzaei, Golrokh, and Hojjat Adeli. "Machine learning techniques for diagnosis of Alzheimer disease, mild cognitive disorder, and other types of dementia." *Biomedical Signal Processing and Control* 72 (2022): 103293.

[25] Brooks, D. J., et al. "Assessment of neuroimaging techniques as biomarkers of the progression of Parkinson's disease." *Experimental Neurology* 184 (2003): 68–79.

[26] Cavalieri, Margherita, Stefan Ropele, Katja Petrovic, Aga Pluta-Fuerst, Nina Homayoon, Christian Enzinger, Anja Grazer et al. "Metabolic syndrome, brain magnetic resonance imaging, and cognition." *Diabetes Care* 33.12 (2010): 2489–2495.

[27] Van De Pol, Laura A., Esther SC Korf, Wiesje M. Van Der Flier, H. Robert Brashear, Nick C. Fox, Frederik Barkhof, and Philip Scheltens. "Magnetic resonance imaging predictors of cognition in mild cognitive impairment." *Archives of Neurology* 64.7 (2007): 1023–1028.

[28] Bonakdarpour, Borna, and Clara Takarabe. "Brain networks, clinical manifestations, and neuroimaging of cognitive disorders: The role of Computed Tomography (CT), Magnetic Resonance Imaging (MRI), Positron Emission Tomography (PET), and Other Advanced Neuroimaging Tests." *Clinics in Geriatric Medicine* 39.1 (2023): 45–65.

[29] Rinne, Juha O., et al. "Cognitive impairment and the brain dopaminergic system in Parkinson disease: [18F] fluorodopa positron emission tomographic study." *Archives of Neurology* 57.4 (2000): 470–475.

[30] Johnson, K. A., et al. "Single photon emission computed tomography perfusion differences in mild cognitive impairment." *Journal of Neurology, Neurosurgery & Psychiatry* 78.3 (2007): 240–247.

[31] Becerra, Judith, Thalia Fernandez, Milene Roca-Stappung, Lourdes Diaz-Comas, Lídice Galán, Jorge Bosch, Marbella Espino, Alma J. Moreno, and Thalía Harmony. "Neurofeedback in healthy elderly human subjects with electroencephalographic risk for cognitive disorder." *Journal of Alzheimer's Disease* 28.2 (2012): 357–367.

[32] Chua, Terence C., Wei Wen, Melissa J. Slavin, and Perminder S. Sachdev. "Diffusion tensor imaging in mild cognitive impairment and Alzheimer's disease: a review." *Current Opinion in Neurology* 21.1 (2008): 83–92.

[33] Mirzaei, Golrokh, and Hojjat Adeli. "Machine learning techniques for diagnosis of Alzheimer disease, mild cognitive disorder, and other types of dementia." *Biomedical Signal Processing and Control* 72 (2022): 103293.

[34] Clarke, Natasha, Thomas R. Barrick, and Peter Garrard. "A comparison of connected speech tasks for detecting early Alzheimer's disease and mild cognitive impairment using natural language processing and machine learning." *Frontiers in Computer Science* 3 (2021): 634360.

[35] Koebel, Kathrin, et al. "Expert insights for designing conversational user interfaces as virtual assistants and companions for older adults with cognitive impairments." Chatbot Research and Design: 5th International Workshop, CONVERSATIONS 2021, Virtual Event, November 23–24, 2021, Revised Selected Papers. Cham: Springer International Publishing, 2022.

[36] Battineni, Gopi, et al. "Artificial intelligence models in the diagnosis of adult-onset dementia disorders: a review." *Bioengineering* 9.8 (2022): 370.

[37] Uddin, Mohammed, Yujiang Wang, and Marc Woodbury-Smith. "Artificial intelligence for precision medicine in neurodevelopmental disorders." *NPJ Digital Medicine* 2.1 (2019): 112.

[38] Koutsouleris, Nikolaos, Christos Davatzikos, Stefan Borgwardt, Christian Gaser, Ronald Bottlender. "Differential diagnosis of schizophrenia and bipolar disorder: comparison of structural MRI and machine learning approaches." *NeuroImage* 93 (2014): 245–255.

[39] Li, X., H. Chen, and F. Pu. "Multi-modal brain imaging feature selection and fusion for Alzheimer's disease diagnosis." *Neurocomputing* 455 (2021): 408–416.

[40] Chopra, Deepti, and Roopal Khurana. *Introduction to machine learning with python.* Bentham Science Publishers, 2023.

[41] Raghupathruni, Kaushik, and Madhavi Dabbiru. "Medical image classification through deep learning." *Computational Intelligence in Data Mining: Proceedings of the International Conference on ICCIDM 2018.* Springer Singapore, 2020.

[42] Cole, James H., Rudra PK Poudel, Dimosthenis Tsagkrasoulis, Matthan WA Caan, Claire Steves, Tim D. Spector, and Giovanni Montana. "Alzheimer's disease neuroimaging initiative. Predicting brain age with deep learning from raw imaging data results in a reliable and heritable biomarker." *NeuroImage* 163 (2018): 115–124.

[43] Ibrahim, Ibrahim Mahmood, and Adnan Mohsin Abdulazeez. "The role of machine learning algorithms for diagnosing diseases." *JASTT* 2.01 (2021): 10–19.

[44] Gandhi, Vaibhav C., and Priyesh P. Gandhi. "A survey-insights of ML and DL in health domain." 2022 International Conference on Sustainable Computing and Data Communication Systems (ICSCDS). IEEE, 2022.

[45] Sánchez Fernández, Iván, and Jurriaan M. Peters. "Machine learning and deep learning in medicine and neuroimaging." *Annals of the Child Neurology Society* 1 (2023): 102–122. https://doi.org/10.1002/cns3.5.

[46] Arbabshirani, Mohammad R., Sergey Plis, Jing Sui, and Vince D. Calhoun. "Single subject prediction of brain disorders in neuroimaging: promises and pitfalls." *NeuroImage* 145 (2017): 137–165.

[47] Rathore, Saima, Mohamad Habes, Muhammad Aksam Iftikhar, Amanda Shacklett, and Christos Davatzikos. "A review on neuroimaging-based classification studies and associated feature extraction methods for Alzheimer's disease and its prodromal stages." *NeuroImage* 155 (2017): 530–548.

CHAPTER 7

Machine Learning and Deep Learning in Deep Brain Stimulation Targeting for Parkinson's Disease

Vikash Agarwal, Swarna M, and Dolly Mushahary

Deep brain stimulation (DBS) has been the most effective procedure for Parkinson's disease (PD) patients. It is an approved surgical procedure for advanced PD, but it is being increasingly used for earlier stages of PD. DBS is used for treating PD especially when levodopa stops being effective. It reduces parkinsonian tremors; further, it correlates to reduced elevation in beta frequency range as involuntary movement does not trigger beta bursting.

Stimulation is supplied through a set of electrodes which are stereotactically implanted (Watt's et al., 2020). The electrodes are connected to a pulse generator, which is implanted subcutaneously and transmits high-frequency electrical impulses to the target area. DBS settings are externally programmed through a hand-held device using an electro-modulator (Follet et al., 2000).

Most challenging part in DBS is the placement of electrodes in exact anatomical location, which indeed maximises efficacy and minimises side effects (Bermdudez et al., 2019). The most common target in DBS for PD patients is the subthalamic nucleus (STN) or globus pallidus interna (GPi), the ventral intermediate (VIM) nucleus of the thalamus for essential tremors, and GPi for dystonia (Watt's et al., 2020, Bermdudez et al., 2019). The success rate of DBS is critically dependent on providing the appropriate required dose of stimulation at the best place within the target location (Boutet et al., 2021). DBS targeting is accomplished with intraoperative image guidance such as 1.5T or 3T magnetic resonance imaging (MRI) or computed tomography (CT) (Watt's et al., 2020, Park et al., 2019).

DOI: 10.1201/9781003264767-7

In terms of target selection for DBS brain of PD, both STN and GPi are considered equally effective in improving the motor symptoms of PD. STN lets a greater medications reduction, while GPi employs a direct anti-dyskinetic effect. VIM nucleus is worth discussing as a further potential target. DBS has always been a preferred surgical target for PD as it has significant long-term benefits for tremor control; at the same time it insufficiently addresses other motor features of PD. DBS in posterior subthalamic area also minimises tremor. Currently the pedunculopontine nucleus remains an investigational target to treat postural instability.

DBS of the GPi is an excellent treatment option for medical refractory dystonia and decreases not only motor impairment but also other impairment (Kupsch et al., 2006; Vidailhet et al., 2005). DBS has been an effective treatment for patients with cervical dystonia or cases that were resistant to botulinum toxin treatment (Volkmann et al., 2014).

Since PD is an asymmetrical disease unilateral pallidotomy has been well known to elicit some bilateral benefits in PD. There is always a question about how DBS for PD can be performed unilaterally, bilaterally, or staged. Unilateral STN-DBS can be proposed for asymmetric patients. There is no evidence that a staged bilateral approach reduces the incidence of DBS-related adverse events (Honey et al., 2016).

Recording neural signals in DBS: In PD, β-band oscillations detected from the basal ganglia correspond to the degree of motor symptoms, such as rigidity and L-3,4-dihydroxyphenylalanine (L-DOPA)-induced dyskinesia, representing a pathophysiological marker of movement disorders that are beyond parkinsonism alone. Presently implantable LFP (local field potential) recording DBS systems are available and they have a non-rechargeable battery which lasts three to five years; these devices have high power consumption that results from LFP acquisition and readouts, limiting the time of use, and lead to earlier replacement of the implantable pulse generator (IPG), a variable that is not supported by patients (Sui et al., 2021). The demand for increasing the longevity of the DBS recording device still remains at the forefront of neural engineering research. This would allow for efficient long-term LFP recordings, for example, to assess the changes of β-band oscillations in response to motor symptoms over time (Sui et al., 2021). PD patients are implanted with a device engineered with rechargeable LFP-sensing and data streaming capacity.

DBS is found to be superior to best medical therapy (BMT) in improving disability, quality of life, and in reducing medication doses, but these benefits need to be compared with the higher risk of serious adverse effects (Bratsos et al., 2018).

Artificial intelligence (AI) in DBS: *Role, introduction, and application*

AI in its broader term can be explained as an application that mimics the cognitive function that machines associate with other human thoughts. AI has a distinguished prospective in medicine and it has been extensively used for understanding neurological diseases and the potential treatments.

AI robustness aides in developing effective treatment for various neurological disorders, such as PD, essential tremors, and dystonia based on data collection (Figure 7.1).

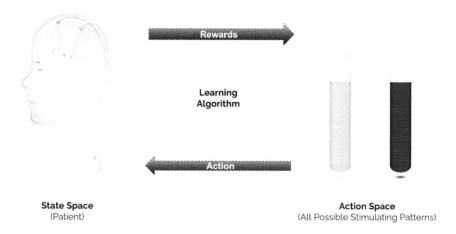

FIGURE 7.1   It explains how the DBS framework can be learned and optimised online with a feedback. State Space represents the patient. Action Space comprises all possible stimulating patterns. A learning algorithm will learn from domain knowledge and history data, then monitor treatment effects (i.e., Reward) and enhance the stimulating pattern (Action) online (Sui et al., 2021).

AI can be represented by two approaches, machine learning (ML) and deep learning (DL). Both are subsets of AI. ML includes algorithms of various types of tasks such as clustering, regression, and classification. ML algorithms need to be trained data rather from particular human programmers. ML comprises building knowledge from gathered patterns in data. The more data we give to the algorithm, the better the algorithm. There are four types of ML algorithms: supervised, semi-supervised, unsupervised, and reinforcement.

ML algorithms are computer-based statistical approaches that can be trained and are able to find common patterns from big amounts of data. In terms of diagnosis of PD, ML models have been applied to a multitude of data modalities, including handwritten patterns, movement, neuroimaging, voice, cerebrospinal fluid (CSF), cardiac scintigraphy, serum and optical coherence tomography (OCT) (Mei et al., 2021). ML also allows for combining different modalities, such as MRI and single-photon emission computed tomography (SPECT) data, in the diagnosis of PD (Mei et al., 2021). By implementing ML methodology, we can determine relevant features that are not traditionally utilised in the clinical diagnosis of PD and depend on these alternative measures to identify PD in preclinical stages or atypical forms.

ML approaches can help clinicians in classifying patients according to several variables at the same time (Landolfi et al., 2021). In a recent study, the promising applications for ML in *DBS candidate selection, programming optimization for better clinical outcomes, facilitation of surgical targeting was demonstrated along with insights into DBS mechanisms* (Watts et al., 2020). ML approaches are commonly used for deriving a diagnostic suggestion, using data collected from multiple sources. Additionally, ML has been applied in real-time, remote monitoring and detection of PD severity, symptoms, and response to therapy

(Belic et al., 2019). Assessing motor and non-motor symptomatology through objective means will allow expansion and robustness of these ML-based decision models.

ML can be used in remote monitoring platforms, which provides an early insight to establish a way to classify symptom severity or cases phenotypes virtually (Watts et al., 2021). Even though there is a limitation to assess potential DBS patients virtually, few studies have provided the efficacy of ML in DBS candidate selection. When potential DBS patients have been recognised, the optimisation of stimulation usually needs frequent and time-consuming programming sessions administered over three to six months from implantation. Effective optimisation of strategic DBS treatment planning using ML has been studied. For instance, computational ML models were developed using preoperative clinical indicators in PD patients treated with STN-DBS. These models were able to accurately stratify PD patients into 60 Hz stimulation or HFS (130–185 Hz) groups *a priori*, offering a unique potential to enhance the utilisation of this therapy based on clinical subtypes (Boutet et al., 2021).

Surgical implantation of electrodes requires exact real-time identification to localise brain region. Presently, imaging with direct MRI-based targeting or coregistration of CT with a 3T MRI are utilised to localise specific anatomic targets STN, GPi, and VIM (Watts et al., 2020). ML techniques are mainly used for microelectrode recording (MER) and to facilitate refined electrode placement (Hariz et al., 2002). Various studies have explored the accuracy of MER; 70% accuracy has been obtained in Cardona et al. studies, which dealt with a retrospective analysis of MER localisation. They weighted traditional ML classifiers with a multi-output Gaussian approach.

In another study, Khosravi et al. (2020, 2019 & 2018) interpreted MERs of electrode trajectories with ML techniques. With the help of 100 DBS subjects they studied, physicians determinations of optimal implantation trajectory's MERs with a deep neural network and achieved an accuracy of 92% in localising specific brain regions, besides they used unsupervised ML techniques on 50 subjects MERs and established the dorsal border of the STN region with 80% accuracy.

ML has also been used in conjunction with the hidden Markov model (HMM) to model surgical planning. Valsky et al. (2020 and 2017) launched a real-time ML classification of the subthalamic border for accurate detection of the STN in DBS surgery. They investigated 58 STN trajectories using a support vector machine (SVM) and attained an accuracy of 97.6%. They used the SVM results to inform an HMM for real-time identification, and this model was tested on an additional 73 trajectories, obtaining a precision of 94%. They also identified the striatopallidal border site to the GPi. They used the same SVM/HMM algorithm for 116 trajectories over three patient types: awake PD patients, lightly anaesthetised genetic, and non-genetic dystonia subjects. Their algorithm had relevant performance for clinical experts for GPi border identification across all patient types considered.

Surgical targeting employs ML to analyse intraoperative signals to increase the targeting of anatomic substrates, fetching immediate clinical relevance as a support tool to assist in surgical planning. Many studies reviewed and used MER signals in classifying or delineating surgical targets to enhance optimal electrode placement; it is important to note that few studies have extensively investigated clinically relevant outcomes relevant to these approaches. Image-based training of surrounding anatomy in ML modelling to enhance surgical target localisation is expanding and showing greater precision and adaptability than current direct (image-guided) or indirect (Talaraich coordinates) methods (Bermudez et al., 2019, Park et al., 2019).

ML is currently employed in the design of DBS systems. Jovanov et al. created a unique adaptive DBS (aDBS) system hardware platform for the real-time optimisation of DBS treatments by generating a genetic algorithm in order to recognise patterns in treatment planning. In recent years technologies like wearables and sensor-based and easy to use systems have been developed for PD patients to assess their symptoms over a prolonged duration. These systems have a great ability to enhance both clinical diagnosis and symptom management.

ML algorithms learnt from data which is large-scale and high-dimensional and gathered from wearable sensors have achieved remarkable success in making accurate predictions for complex problems in which human skill has been required to date, but they are challenging to evaluate and apply without a basic understanding of the underlying logic on which they are based (Kubota et al., 2016).

This technology has the potential to significantly improve both clinical diagnosis and management in PD and the conduct of clinical studies. However, the large-scale, high-dimensional character of the data captured by these wearable sensors requires sophisticated signal processing and ML algorithms to transform it into scientifically and clinically meaningful information. Such algorithms that "learn" from data have shown remarkable success in making accurate predictions for complex problems in which human skill has been required to date, but they are challenging to evaluate and apply without a basic understanding of the underlying logic on which they are based (Kubota et al., 2016).

Application of wearables for aDBS will rely heavily on ML approaches for distinguishing symptoms from voluntary movements (Habets et al., 2018). Adaptive DBS has a significant scope of clinical impact on a patient's quality of life. LFPs and/or wearable sensors serve as robust measurement instruments for the classification of specific behavioural tasks and for assessing severity or tremor. However, a large portion of these studies utilised assessments obtained in a clinical setting. Further work is required to identify motor control symptoms in real-world environments. Tremor detection using wearable sensors appears to be one of the closest methods for application in the clinical field. Additionally, the development of HMMs that accurately describe a DBS would have a great impact on strategic treatment planning. To that end, dynamic treatment planning would require a further assessment as to the practicality of adaptively tuning DBS parameters (Watts et al., 2020).

Use of ML assisted diagnosis of PD results in high potential for a more systematic clinical decision-making system, while application of novel biomarkers will increase access to PD diagnosis at an earlier stage. Therefore, ML-based approaches have significant prospective to provide clinicians with additional tools to screen, detect, or diagnose PD (Mei et al., 2021).

DL in DBS: *DL-based targeting techniques*

DL is a branch or a subset of ML that deals with algorithms inspired by the structure and function of the brain, called artificial neural networks. DL uses Artificial Neural Networks

(ANN) comprising many layers (e.g., >6) and is commonly considered as a more advanced method of ML, which is able to perform more detailed analysis, combining more data and able to represent higher levels of abstraction. Each node receives information from other nodes and the outputs from those nodes are weighted (Currie et al., 2019). The training phase has the best outcomes with a large data set. Big data in medical imaging plays an important role in providing large, reliable training data for ML and DL algorithms to learn from. DL describes the depth or number of layers in the ANN and is generally associated with CNNs to identify and extract features directly from images (Currie et al., 2019). In sum, the DL model is trained using a large amount of labelled data and a neural network architecture that learns features directly from the data without the need for manual feature extraction.

Image-guided surgery is regarded as a potential application of DL (Naylor, 2018; Mehrtash et al., 2017). Clinical approaches to surgical planning for DBS depend on imaging interpretation and processing, including MRI-based direct targeting and image fusion techniques using coregistration with CT and 1.5T and 3T MRI (Park et al., 2019).

Frequently quoted applications of DL in medical imaging applications are as follows: object detection (e.g., location of a lesion), object segmentation (e.g., lesion contouring), and object classification (e.g., malignant vs. benign lesion) (Currie et al., 2019).

Direct targeting using DL-based image interpretation can be possible when target visualisation is achieved with sufficient resolution. Later, electrophysiologic information, including MER and intraoperative stimulation effects, can be considered for final decisions regarding electrode positions (Park et al., 2019 & 2017).

Semantic segmentation results in pixel-wise image classification into predetermined classes, for example, anatomical structures. It combines classification information ("what") and location information ("where") from image data. Semantic segmentation can classify and identify the margins of multiple types of objects (Shelhamer et al., 2017).

Recent convolutional neural network segmentation studies have not been optimised for the STN or red nucleus but instead for basal ganglia structures or the striatum only (Park et al., 2019). Therefore, DL-based semantic segmentation of the STN and red nucleus is not well investigated. Thus, the current state-of-the-art methods for STN and red nucleus semantic segmentation are non-DL methods (Kim et al., 2019; Shamir et al., 2019).

Automatic targeting methods for DBS have significant clinical benefits and may be non-inferior to manual methods. In spite of that, the clinical application of automatic targeting methods is still under further investigation (Pallavaram et al., 2015). Compared to other automatic methods, widespread applicability may have been limited due to the high variability of the STN anatomy (Naylor, 2018). DL-based semantic segmentation shows unambiguous adaptability to considerable variations in STN shape, which enables real-world clinical application (Park et al., 2019).

Dice coefficient is a statistic used to measure the similarity of two samples. Non-DL adaptive algorithms, as well as semantic segmentation studies of the basal ganglia and brainstem structure, have used simpler image features than DL (Shamir et al., 2019). It follows that DL may be more adaptive to anatomical variation and better at generalisation using more abstractive features. Thus, the final segmentation accuracy may be higher when DL is used.

There are two types of DL-based targeting techniques: direct and indirect. Direct learning refers to hard facts logically implied by the data. For instance, given a data base on MRI scans of patients with PD, we could inquire who has shown different stages of PD and how their progression looks like. DL-based targeting method is highly objective, extractable, consistent and can be evaluated compared to manual methods. DL DBS can aid in standardisation of targeting locations in multi-centre clinical trials involving different surgeons (Park et al., 2019).

Direct targets are based on MRI anatomical structure margins (Park et al., 2019). Since this DL-based targeting relies on MRI anatomical structure margins, it can be regarded as a kind of MRI-based direct targeting method (Bejjani et al., 2000).

Indirect learning refers to inferences drawn from the data. Indirect targeting is based on Talairach coordinates (brain in three-dimensional space). For instance, given a data base of MRI scans of patients with movement disorder, we could identify clusters of patients who showed certain anatomical substrates and use those correlations to predict other patients' possible structural variability during the progression of the movement disorder, even if the patient had not showcased it yet. Usually, indirect targets were manually computed and exhibited for comparison reasons.

Localisation of DBS targets can differ among surgeons and DBS centres and best locations are controversial. A few surgeons target the centre of the STN, while others target more medial sites, medial-posterior sites, or other locations (Park et al., 2019). Certainly, individual surgeons may not be consistent in this regard. Thus, the location of a quantified point or line (e.g., 1 mm lateral from the medial border of the STN) may vary among individual surgeons when targeting is manually applied. Nevertheless, when similar DL algorithm models and input images are applied, targeting is totally identical and can be standardised without any subjective differences.

REFERENCES

Bejjani, B.P., Dormont, D., Pidoux, B., Yelnik, J., Damier, P., Arnulf, I., et al. Bilateral subthalamic stimulation for Parkinson's disease by using three- dimensional stereotactic magnetic resonance imaging and electrophysiological guidance. *J. Neurosurg.* **2000**, *92*, 615–625. doi: 10.3171/jns.2000.92.4.0615

Bermdudez, C., Rodriguez, S., Huo, Y., Hainline, A., Li, R., Shults, R., Haese, P., Konrad, P., Dawant, M., and Landman, B. Towards machine learning prediction of deep brain stimulation (DBS) intra-operative efficacy maps. *Medical Imaging Image Processing.* **2019**, 1094922.

Boutet, A., Madhavan, R., Elias, G., Joel, S., Gramer, R., Ranjan, M., Paramanandam,V., Xu, D., Germann, J., Loh, A., Kalia, S., Hodaie, M., Li, B., Prasad, S., Coblentz, A., Munhoz, R., Ashe, J., Kucharczyk, W., Fasano, A., and Lozano, A. Predicting optimal deep brain stimulation parameters for Parkinson's disease using functional MRI and machine learning. *Nat Commun.* **2021**, *12*, 3043.

Bratsos, P.S., Tarpons, D., and Saleh, N.S. Efficacy and safety of deep brain stimulation in the treatment of Parkinson's disease: A systematic review and meta-analysis of randomized controlled trials. *Cureus.* **2018**, *10*(10), e3474. doi: 10.7759/cureus.3474

Belic, M., Bobic, V., Badža, M., Šolaja, N., Đuric-Jovicˇic, M., and Kostic, V.S. Artificial intelligence for assisting diagnostics and assessment of Parkinson's disease—A review. *Clin. Neurol. Neurosurg.* **2019**, *184*, 105442.

Bermudez, C., Rodriguez, W., Huo, Y., Hainline, A.E., Li, R., Shults, R., D'Haese, P.D., Konrad, P.E., Dawant, B.M., and Landman, B.A. Towards machine learning prediction of deep brain stimulation (DBS) intra-operative efficacy maps. In *Proceedings of the Medical Imaging 2019: Image Processing*, San Diego, CA, USA, 16–21 February 2019; p. 1094922.

Currie, G. Intelligent imaging: Artificial intelligence augmented nuclear medicine. *J. Nucl Med. Technol.* **2019**, *47*, 217–222.

Follett, K.A. The surgical treatment of Parkinson's disease. *Annu. Rev. Med.* **2000**, *51*, 135–147. doi: 10.1146/annurev.med.51.1.135

Hariz, M.I. Safety and risk of microelectrode recording in surgery for movement disorders. *Stereotact. Funct. Neurosurg.* **2002**, *78*, 146–157.

Habets, J.G.V., Heijmans, M., Kuijf. M.L., Janssen, M.L.F., Temel, Y., and Kubben, P.L. An update on adaptive deep brain stimulation in Parkinson's disease. *Mov. Disord.* **2018** Dec, *33*(12), 1834–1843. doi: 10.1002/mds.115. Epub 2018 Oct 24. PMID: 30357911; PMCID: PMC6587997.

Khosravi, M., Atashzar, S.F., Gilmore, G., Jog, M.S., and Patel, R.V. Electrophysiological signal processing for intraoperative localization of subthalamic nucleus during deep brain stimulation surgery. In *Proceedings of the 2018 IEEE Global Conference on Signal and Information Processing (GlobalSIP)*, Anaheim, CA, USA, 26–28 November 2018; pp. 424–428.

Khosravi, M., Atashzar, S.F., Gilmore, G., Jog, M.S., and Patel, R.V. Unsupervised clustering of microelectrophysiological signals for localization of subthalamic nucleus during DBS Surgery. In *Proceedings of the 2019 9th International IEEE/EMBS Conference on Neural Engineering (NER)*, San Francisco, CA, USA, 20–23 March 2019; pp. 17–20.

Khosravi, M., Atashzar, S.F., Gilmore, G., Jog, M.S., and Patel, R.V. Intraoperative localization of STN during DBS surgery using a data-driven model. *IEEE J. Transl. Eng. Health Med.* **2020**, *8*, 1–9.

Kim, J., Duchin, Y., Shamir, R.R., Patriat, R., Vitek, J., Harel, N., et al. Automatic localization of the subthalamic nucleus on patient-specific clinical MRI by incorporating 7 T MRI and machine learning: Application in deep brain stimulation. *Hum. Brain Mapp.* **2019**, *40*, 679–698. doi: 10.1002/hbm.24404

Kupsch, A., Benecke, R., Müller, J., Trottenberg, T., Schneider, G.H., Poewe, W., et al. Deep-brain stimulation for dystonia study group. Pallidal deep-brain stimulation in primary generalized or segmental dystonia. *N. Engl. J. Med.* **2006,** *355*, 1978–1990. doi: 10.1056/NEJMoa063618

Kubota, K.J., Chen, J.A., and Little, M.A. Machine learning for large-scale wearable sensor data in Parkinson's disease: Concepts, promises, pit- falls, and futures. *Mov. Disord.* **2016**, *31*, 1314–1326.

Landolfi, A., Ricciardi, C., Donisi, L., Cesarelli, G., Troisi, J., Vitale, C., … & Amboni, M. Machine learning approaches in Parkinson's Disease. *Curr. Med. Chem.* **2021**, *28*(32), 6548–6568.

Mei, J., Desrosiers, C. and Frasnelli, J. Machine learning for the diagnosis of Parkinson's Disease: A review of literature. *Front. Aging. Neurosci.* **2021**, *13*, 633752. doi: 10.3389/fnagi.2021.633752

Naylor, C.D. On the prospects for a (deep) learning health care system. *JAMA.* **2018**, *320*, 1099–1100.

Park, S.C., Cha, J.H., Lee, S., Jang, W., Lee, C.S., and Lee, J.K. Deep learning-based deep brain stimulation targeting and clinical applications. *Front. Neurosci.* **2019**, *13*, 1128.

Park, S.C., Lee, C.S., Kim, S.M., Choi, E.J., and Lee, J.K. Comparison of the stereotactic accuracies of function-guided deep brain stimulation, calculated using multitrack target locations geometrically inferred from three-dimensional trajectory rotations, and of magnetic resonance imaging-guided deep brain stimulation and outcomes. *World Neurosurg.* **2017**, *98*, 734.e7–749. e7. doi: 10.1016/ j.wneu.2016.11.046

Pallavaram, S., D'haese, P.F., Lake, W., Konrad, P.E., Dawant, B.M., and Neimat, J.S. Fully automated targeting using nonrigid image registration matches accuracy and exceeds precision of best manual approaches to subthalamic deep brain stimulation targeting in Parkinson disease. *Neurosurgery.* **2015**, *76*, 756–765. doi: 10.1227/NEU.0000000000000714

Shelhamer, E., Long, J., and Darrell, T. Fully convolutional networks for semantic segmentation. *IEEE Trans. Pattern Anal. Mach Intell.* **2017**, *39*, 640–651. doi: 10.1109/TPAMI.2016.2572683

Shamir, R.R., Duchin, Y., Kim, J., Patriat, R., Marmor, O., Bergman, H., et al. Microelectrode recordings validate the clinical visualization of subthalamic-nucleus based on 7T magnetic resonance imaging and machine learning for deep brain stimulation surgery. *Neurosurgery.* **2019**, *84*, 749–757. doi: 10.1093/neuros/nyy212

Sui, Y., Tian, Y., Ko, W.K.G., Wang, Z., Jia, F., Horn, A., De Ridder, D., Choi, K.S., Bari, A.A., Wang, S., Hamani, C., Baker, K.B., Machado, A.G., Aziz, T.Z., Fonoff, E.T., Kühn, A.A., Bergman, H., Sanger, T., Liu, H., Haber, S.N. and Li, L. Deep brain stimulation initiative: Toward innovative technology, new disease indications, and approaches to current and future clinical challenges in neuromodulation therapy. *Front. Neurol.* **2021**, *11*, 597451. doi: 10.3389/fneur.2020.597451

Valsky, D., Marmor-Levin, O., Deffains, M., Eitan, R., Blackwell, K.T., Bergman, H., and Israel, Z. Stop! border ahead: Automatic detection of subthalamic exit during deep brain stimulation surgery. *Mov. Disord.* **2017**, *32*, 70–79.

Valsky, D., Blackwell, K.T., Tamir, I., Eitan, R., Bergman, H., and Israel, Z. Real-time machine learning classification of pallidal borders during deep brain stimulation surgery. *J. Neural Eng.* **2020**, *17*, 016021.

Vidailhet, M., Vercueil, L., Houeto, J.L., Krystkowiak, P., Benabid, A.L., Cornu, P., et al. French stimulation du pallidum interne dans la dystonie (SPIDY) study group. Bilateral deep-brain stimulation of the globus pallidus in primary generalized dystonia. *N. Engl. J. Med.* **2005**, *352*, 459–467. doi: 10.1056/NEJMoa042187.

Volkmann, J., Mueller, J., Deuschl, G., Kühn, A.A., Krauss, J.K., Poewe, W., et al. DBS study group for dystonia. Pallidal neurostimulation in patients with medication-refractory cervical dystonia: A randomised, sham-controlled trial. *Lancet. Neurol.* **2014**, *13*, 875–884. doi: 10.1016/S1474-4422(14)70143-7

Watts, J., Khojandi, A., Shylo, O., and Ramdhani, R. Machine learning's application in deep brain stimulation for Parkinson's disease: A review. *Brain Sci.* **2020**, *10,* 809.

Index

Note: **Bold** page numbers refer to tables; *italic* page numbers refer to figures.

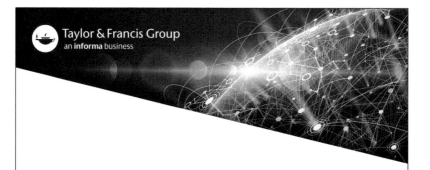